the MINDFULNESS journal

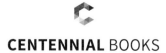

CENTENNIAL BOOKS

CENTENNIAL BOOKS

the MINDFULNESS journal

The Ultimate Guide To Well-Being

BY ANNE MARIE O'CONNOR

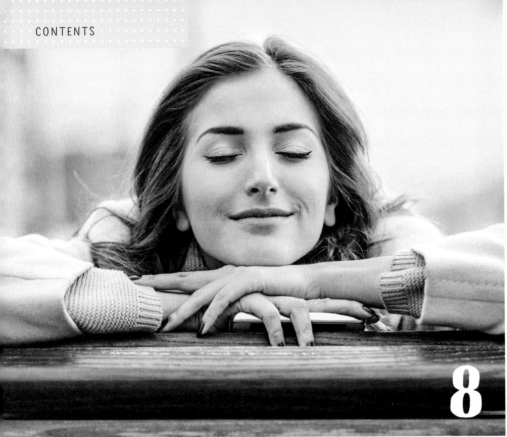

8

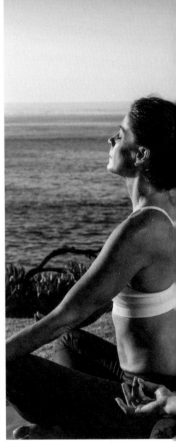

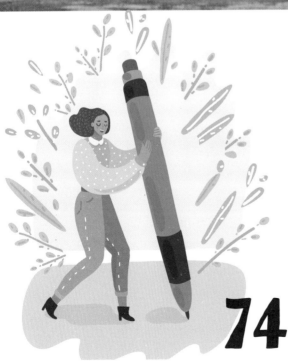

74

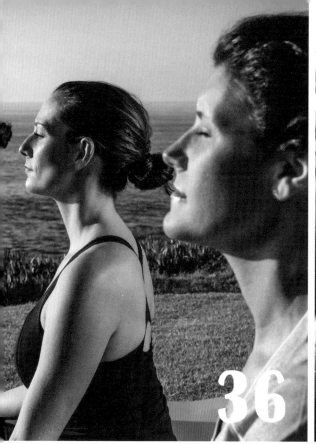

36

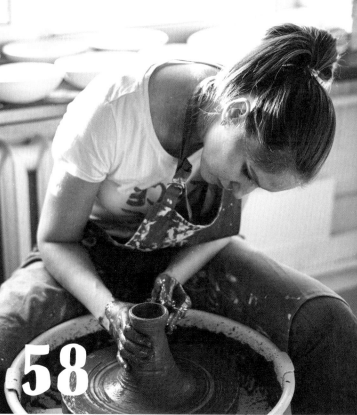

58

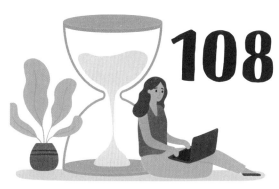

108

live your
BEST LIFE

By learning to become more mindful,
we can decrease our stress levels, feel happier
and focus on what's really important.

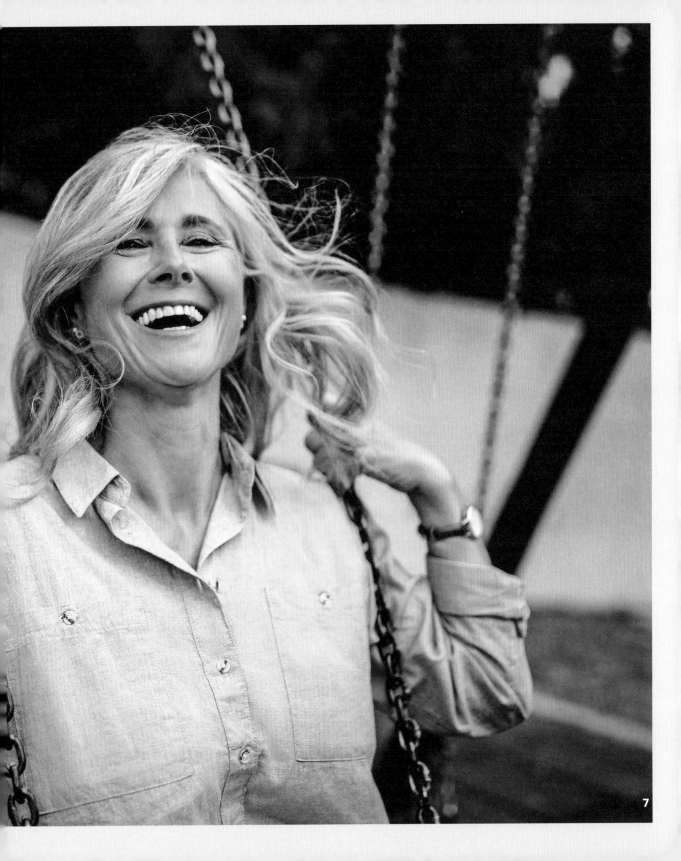

THE MAGIC OF MINDFULNESS

Scientists are now confirming what Buddhists have believed for centuries: Mindfulness has the power to transform nearly every aspect of your life.

Confession: Before I delved into the world of mindfulness, I thought of it as something I didn't have the energy for. The idea of obsessing over every bite of my salad or being laser-focused on my kids 24/7 felt, well, exhausting. And when my "stress alarm" went off, there's no way I'd remember to take calming breaths, especially when junk food was in reach.

But I quickly learned that being mindful isn't as arduous as I'd thought. "It's basically anything you're doing that you're paying attention to—without judgment, ruminating or worrying," explains Julie Potiker, a Mindful Self-Compassion teacher and author of *Life Falls Apart, But You Don't Have To: Mindful Methods for Staying Calm in the Midst of Chaos*.

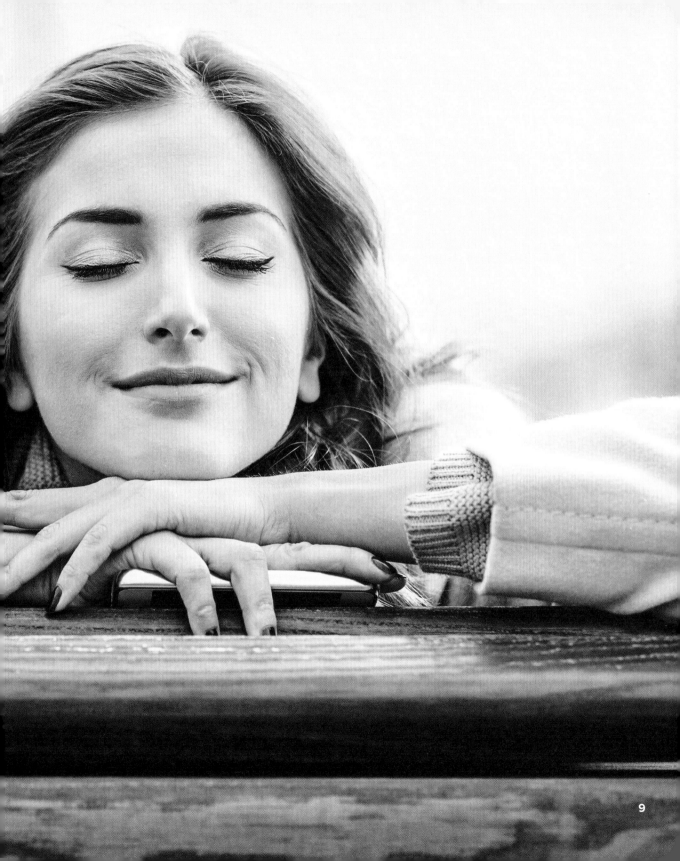

Another way to look at it: "When we're not being mindful, we're just going through the motions of life," says Suzie Carmack, PhD, a well-being expert and author of three books, including *Genius Breaks: Optimize Your Workday Performance and Well-Being.* "Mindfulness techniques—meditation, mindful eating, mindful movement, etc.—are all different ways to practice being more compassionate in our day-to-day living. You learn to be more strategic about how you live your life and support those you care about to do the same."

When it comes to living a truly mindful life, Carmack says it's really all about balancing the internal distractions (our worries, doubts and feelings that might arise unexpectedly) with the external stuff (hello, constant ping of technology). "Ultimately, if we ignore distractions or difficulties, we're not being mindful, either. So it's not all 'perfect.' To me, it boils down to three things: awareness, intention and compassion." (Not having to be perfect? That's a relief!).

HOW MINDFULNESS BECAME A MOVEMENT

Although mindfulness is a concept rooted in Hindu and Buddhist contemplative traditions that go back thousands of years, these days there's nothing "new-agey" about it. In 1979, Jon Kabat-Zinn, PhD, a professor of medicine at the University of Massachusetts, founded the Mindfulness-Based Stress Reduction (MBSR) clinic—and then the Center for Mindfulness in Medicine, Health Care, and Society—thus giving mindfulness credibility in the medical world.

"It was stripped from its origins and moved into a Western medical center and was mainstreamed," Potiker says. Carmack concurs with that idea: "I admire how Kabat-Zinn pulled mindfulness down into a very practical approach that could be replicated, so that it was no longer this abstract concept that was too 'woo-woo.' He also held it up to the light of scientific rigor so that even people who were skeptical were shown that yes, this really works."

A MULTITUDE OF POSITIVE BENEFITS

Thanks to the efforts of Kabat-Zinn and a handful of other influencers—including Jack Kornfield, Sharon Salzberg and Joseph Goldstein, who together opened the Insight Meditation Society in 1975—the scientific world took notice. "We're at a tipping point," Potiker says. "There have been hundreds of research papers published on MBSR in the past 10 years."

With this stream of research, came validation—and acceptance. "It's amazing to see how mindfulness-based interventions are having positive effects in various areas, such as anxiety, depression, emotion regulation, relationships and the ability to maintain healthy habits," Potiker notes.

And the list of benefits goes on—and on. Mindful people are more likely to have lower blood pressure, as reported in a 2013 study in *Psychosomatic Medicine: Journal of Biobehavioral Medicine.* A 2018 study published in the journal *PAIN* reported that more mindful people tend to have a higher pain threshold.

In 2016, scientists from Case Western Reserve University in Ohio discovered that a more mindful corporate culture improved overall employee focus, stress levels and relationships. And a 2017 study out of the University of Pennsylvania found that mindful individuals made better health choices, such as those around diet and exercise.

In 2018, researchers from Penn State University concluded that mindful movement—specifically walking—eased stress and anxiety in students; the more mindfully they walked, the bigger the benefits. And research in the journal *Body Image* linked mindfulness to better body image and regulation of internal body cues, such as hunger.

So if the advantages are so vast—and so important in this day and age, when the world is moving at such a rapid pace—why aren't more of us adopting a more mindful lifestyle?

EVEN A LITTLE GOES A LONG WAY

Well, for one, there's a case of misconstruing the core essence of mindfulness (see the first paragraph of

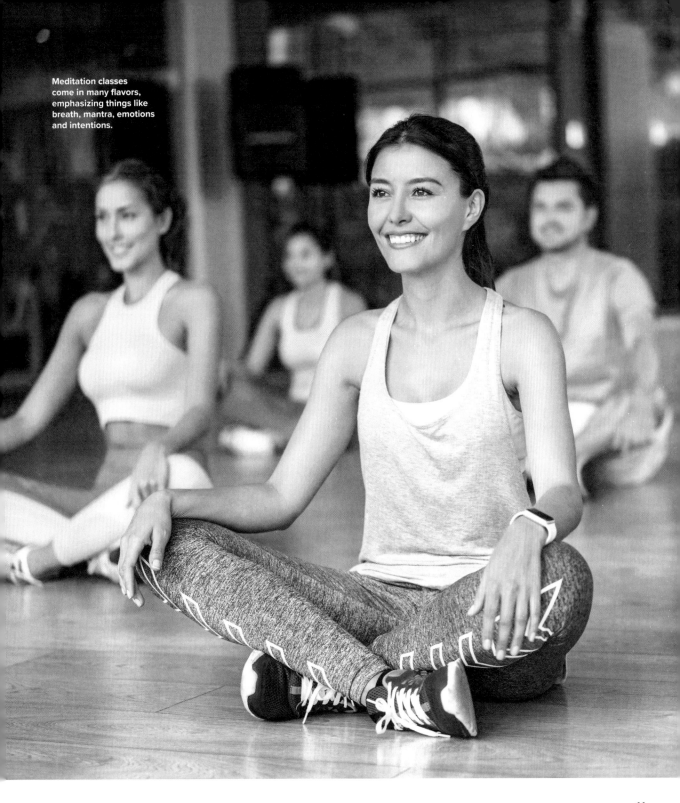

Meditation classes come in many flavors, emphasizing things like breath, mantra, emotions and intentions.

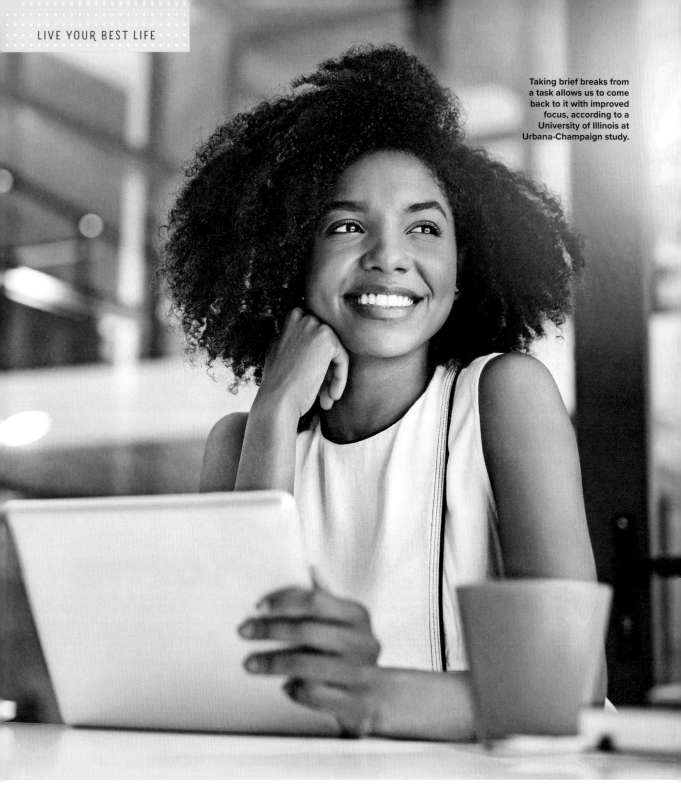

Taking brief breaks from a task allows us to come back to it with improved focus, according to a University of Illinois at Urbana-Champaign study.

this story). Carmack, too, once shared my sentiments, believing that mindfulness wasn't worth her time. "I used to run out before the meditation part of yoga class," she recalls with a laugh. "I felt like, hey, I've got work to do, kids to take care of, I'm out of here." (Now, as a teacher to other wellness professionals, from health coaches to yoga teachers to corporate leaders in her Center for Well-Being Education module, she emphasizes that meditation is one of the most important parts of their day.)

"Meditation uses a prompt [such as your breath, a word, a phrase, or movement like tai chi] to anchor the mind and help people get mindful; it's a building block for mindfulness," says Potiker. "It slows everything down and enables you to get in touch with what's going on in your body, which is important because we're not just living in our brains."

Even a little meditation goes a long way, she points out. "I want people to meditate 10 minutes a day, leading up to 20 minutes, and then they can do mindfulness activities in daily life and have more of an awareness of their thoughts, feelings and emotions as they come up, pass and fall away."

But meditation is just one technique under the rather large umbrella of mindfulness. "Mindfulness is your own dance with your consciousness," Carmack reasons. "Meditation is one type of dance, but there are many. I've seen people who have a very rigorous meditation practice and are still working on being more mindful—and vice versa. And you know what? It's all good. The minute that any of us starts thinking that there's only one way to do it, or one way to get there, we've missed out on the joy. Each of us has our own dance for this life—and we are the only one who gets to truly lead it."

FIND WHAT WORKS FOR YOU

● When it comes to mindfulness, one thing is clear: There's no one-size-fits-all solution. Potiker is a firm believer in loading up your tool box with a hefty set of tools, and then mixing and matching them as needed. "There's enough data to say that these practices can help you in these five or 10 ways and why," she says, "so let's see what happens. Try seeing what works for you."

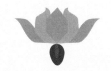

DON'T FORGET TO BREATHE

Breathing might be one of the most simple, yet most effective, strategies for helping to reel in chaotic thoughts. "Breathing drops your blood pressure and heart rate," mindfulness teacher Julie Potiker explains. "It takes you from your sympathetic nervous system to your parasympathetic. It helps to down-regulate cortisol and adrenaline when you're in fight-or-flight mode and need to chill." Play around with the following breathing techniques to help turn your mood around.

→ **BREATHE IN FOR 4, HOLD FOR 5, THEN EXHALE FOR 6** "The counting is an anchor for your attention that diminishes the chatter and takes you away from something stressful," Potiker says.

→ **TRY A LONGER INHALE—OR EXHALE** "Breathing in for a little longer can be very invigorating for some," author Suzie Carmack says, "while a longer exhale can be calming."

→ **BREATHE IN AND OUT EVENLY** "An equal ratio of inhale to exhale can help focus your mind," suggests Carmack.

→ **LINK BREATH WITH WORDS** "Breathe in the word 'grate' and exhale the word 'full,' imagining that you're breathing in a perfume of gratitude," she says.

And the more you pull out your mindful techniques, the easier choosing the right one for a particular situation will be. "When you practice a lot, you get your go-tos," Potiker adds. Maybe it's meditation, journaling, a breathing technique (check out the sidebar, above) or even "putting your

FIVE WAYS TO FEEL MORE PRESENT...IN MINUTES

Need to calm down—and fast? Try these quick yet powerful techniques.

➜ **PUT ON SOME MUSIC** "If you're listening to music and really allowing it to move you, you can look at that as a mindfulness, meditative activity," instructor Julie Potiker says. "The point is that you're not worrying or ruminating."

➜ **TAKE A BREAK** "Sometimes we need to pull over from the pace of life and give our brain a reboot, so we can get back into a proactive state," Suzie Carmack, PhD, says. "Our entire stress response is built on our perception of threat, so taking these breaks is important." A few ideas: Close your eyes, call a friend, get up and move—doing the last of these can increase your creativity by as much as 60 percent, notes Carmack.

➜ **REFRAME YOUR STORY** Pick a "chakra of communication theme" for the day—a practice that Carmack came up with. "Choose either respect, gratitude, commitment, courage, kindness, insight, community or consciousness, and morph it into a positive self-talk statement such as, 'I'm going to be courageous,' or 'I'm going to be as kind to myself as I am to others.' The themes are meant to help you reframe the story you are telling yourself in chaotic moments, so that you have a new way to experience the moment and consciously choose to stop self-catastrophizing thoughts."

➜ **LOVE THYSELF** Loving-kindness is a type of meditation that "invites you to expand your ability to have compassion for yourself and others, including those whom you find off-putting," Potiker explains. She suggests using a mantra like, "May you be safe, may you be healthy, may you live with ease." Adds Potiker, "I run through sets of these phrases while waiting in the airport security line, and by the time I get to the TSA employee, I'm radiating love, which gets picked up and mirrored automatically. Imagine having that positive juju brightening up so many lives that day!"

➜ **REWIRE YOUR BRAIN FOR JOY** "Whenever you find yourself experiencing something joyful, pause for a moment, breathe and really let it sink in," Potiker suggests. "That marinating-in-the-good helps rewire your brain for happiness and resilience. Then when you're experiencing stress, retrieve this joyful memory to help break the discursive loop."

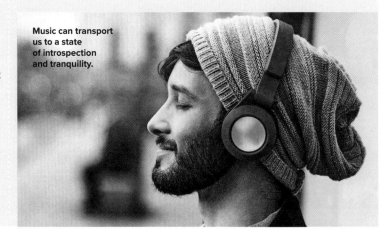

Music can transport us to a state of introspection and tranquility.

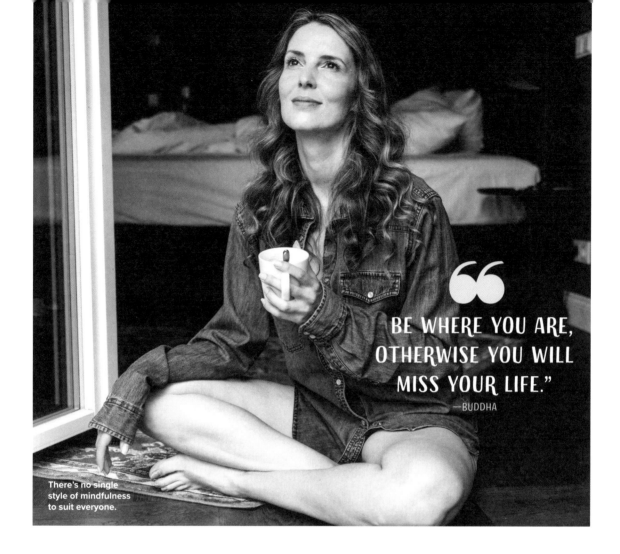

66

BE WHERE YOU ARE,
OTHERWISE YOU WILL
MISS YOUR LIFE."
—BUDDHA

There's no single
style of mindfulness
to suit everyone.

hand on your heart and using that soothing touch to help down-regulate cortisol and adrenaline, and release oxytocin."

The key, per Potiker, is to throw a bunch of techniques at the wall and see what works for you. "The proof is in the pudding. Maybe you'll notice that you seem less reactive or are nicer, or that your relationship skills have improved."

When it comes to being more mindful in daily life, it's simple. "It could be having the first few sips of your morning beverage mindfully," Potiker suggests. "I feel the warm mug in my hands, look at the color of my coffee as I stir in my creamer, smell the delicious aroma and then take my first mindful

sip. The whole time, I am focusing my attention on the experience, not my to-do list. Before I know it, I have given my brain a two-minute break from worrying and ruminating!" (For more fast and easy ways to practice mindfulness, see opposite page.)

No matter what works best for you, be careful not to put too much pressure on yourself, adds Carmack. "We have this long list of things we 'should' be doing. Let's reinforce the idea that being mindful is not a 'should'— it's a 'could' and a 'want to,' because it helps us remember the truth inside, no matter what's outside. Ultimately, it's about connecting with that joy."

—*Amanda Altman*

THE SCIENCE OF BEING IN THE MOMENT

Mindfulness isn't some woo-woo thing for Buddhist monks and the Goop crowd; it offers tangible, research-backed benefits for everyone.

Every day, scientists are discovering more and more health benefits from mindfulness. Whether it's meditation, yoga or journaling, these practices can help you reduce stress, enhance memory and concentration, boost your immune system, and help you feel calmer and live a more content life in general. "Mindfulness is such a powerful tool for both mind and body because it really forces you to focus on where you are at the present moment," explains Alice Domar, PhD, executive director of the Domar Center for Mind/Body Health and the director of mind/body services at Boston IVF in Boston. Here's a look at some of the evidence.

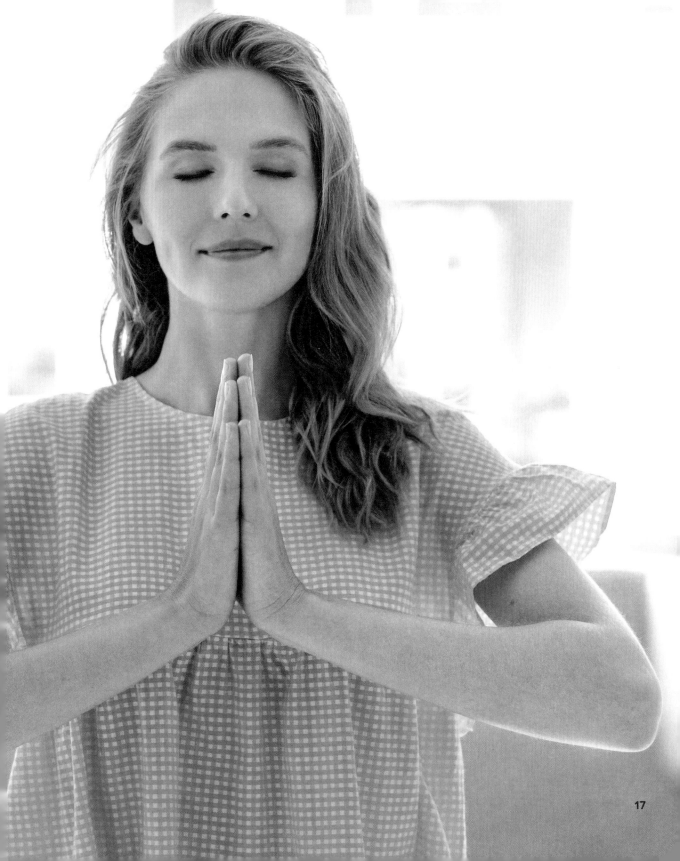

ENHANCES MEMORY AND CONCENTRATION

• People who took a four-week online mindfulness course, where they learned to focus on their breathing and body sensations, performed much better on memory tests than those who took an online creative writing course, a study in *Brain Imaging and Behavior* found. They also experienced an increase in their hippocampus, the part of the brain associated with memory and concentration. "[These therapies] help reduce stress and inflammation, which are both toxic to the brain," explains Thomas Wisniewski, MD, director of the Center for Cognitive Neurology at New York University Medical Center. They may also enhance production of brain-derived neurotrophic growth factor, a protein that stimulates connections between neurons.

IMPROVES YOUR HEART HEALTH

• Mindfulness practices such as meditation appear to help reduce your risk of heart disease, according to a 2017 scientific statement published in the *Journal of the American Heart Association.* In it, experts reviewed dozens of studies published over the past two decades; they found evidence that meditation aided in lowering blood pressure, decreasing blood glucose levels and improving blood flow to the heart. In addition, meditation helped with smoking cessation, which is also beneficial to cardiovascular health.

PROMOTES BETTER SLEEP

• Research suggests mindfulness may make it easier to get your z's. After just six weeks, people who practiced mindfulness meditation improved sleep scores by 2.8 points—more than twice as much as a group who only practiced sleep-hygiene methods such as eliminating napping and establishing a relaxing regular bedtime routine, according to a 2015 study in *JAMA Internal Medicine.* "So much of insomnia is tied to stress: People can't fall asleep because their minds are racing," explains Alexander Mauskop, MD, FAAN, director of the New York Headache Center in NYC. "But by really focusing on your breathing, and closing your mind to all other thoughts, you're creating an atmosphere where you can relax and fall asleep."

IMPROVES YOUR MOOD

• Mindfulness-based cognitive therapy, which trains the brain to deal with negative emotions using meditation techniques, is just as effective as antidepressant drugs, a 2016 study in *JAMA Psychiatry* found. And you get bonus points if you add some exercise into the mix. Women who suffered from post-traumatic stress disorder who did a combination of meditation and aerobic exercise for one hour twice a week over six weeks significantly reduced symptoms, according to research published in 2018 in *Frontiers in Neuroscience.*

RELIEVES HEADACHES

• When adult migraine sufferers took part in a mindfulness-based stress-reduction program that combined meditation and yoga for 45 minutes five days of the week, they experienced fewer and significantly shorter migraines (almost three hours shorter) than those who didn't do the intervention, according to a 2014 study in the journal *Headache.* "Meditation stops the brain from being overactive, which may in turn slow down the pain messages bombarding your brain cells," explains Mauskop.

BOOSTS YOUR IMMUNE SYSTEM

• Sure, you know that eating a healthy diet, exercising and getting enough sleep helps keep your immune system in tiptop shape, but mindfulness can help keep you from coming down with a cold or the flu, too. This is because stress itself dampens immunity by forcing your body to churn out stress hormones such as cortisol, which suppresses your immune system, explains Bruce Rabin, MD, PhD, emeritus professor of preventative medicine at the University of Pittsburgh. It also ramps up inflammation in your body, which in turn can dial down immunity. A 2016 UCLA review of 20 randomized control trials published in the *Annals of the New York Academy of Science* found that mindfulness meditation reduced markers of inflammation and increased the number of CD4 cells (a type of immune-system cell). So not only will an apple a day keep the doctor away—so will a yoga or meditation practice.

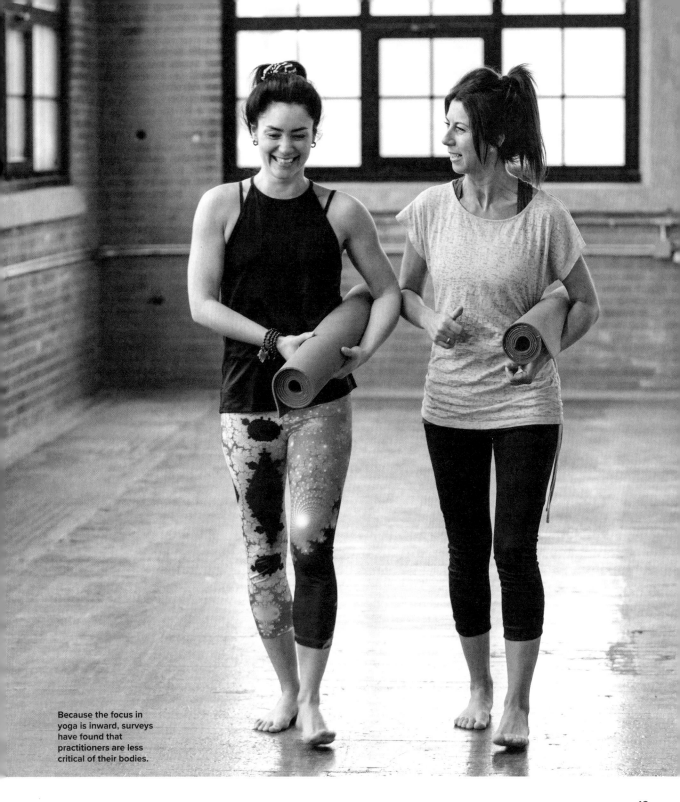

Because the focus in yoga is inward, surveys have found that practitioners are less critical of their bodies.

TAKING THE FIRST STEPS

It's easy to get started on your mindfulness journey. Here's how.

You don't have to move to a monastery in Tibet or do hours of yoga a day to reap the benefits of mindfulness. Plus, its positive effects on your brain and body happen fairly quickly. When people meditated every day for eight weeks, they showed changes in parts of their brain such as the hippocampus, cortex and amygdala similar to those who had been meditating for years, according to a 2016 study in *Brain and Cognition*. "It's never too late to start, and you don't have to do much to see results," says researcher Bruce Rabin, MD. Some things to keep in mind:

→ YOU DON'T NEED TO SIT STILL

If you think mindfulness requires sitting upright in a chair chanting *om*, relax. There are plenty of ways to move around and practice mindfulness at the same time. Try a mind-body activity like yoga or tai chi, which incorporate mindfulness with their emphasis on slow movements, controlled breathing and focus. It can also be any sort of exercise that's repetitive, adds mind/body expert Alice Domar, PhD, like running, swimming laps or even walking. Just focus on the present moment—the feeling of

your arms moving through water, or the sound your feet make as they hit the pavement—and if your mind keeps wandering, pick a sound to repeat over and over in your mind, like "peace" or "om." Journaling, a gratitude practice, volunteering and even bird-watching can also be mindful activities.

→ START SMALL

If you're new to mindfulness, begin with short, three- to five-minute sessions, advises Domar. One exercise to try: a body scan. While sitting or lying down, take a few slow, deep breaths, focusing on your forehead. Ask yourself: Is there any muscle tension as I exhale? Can I relax my forehead muscles? Then move down to your eyes. Are they squeezed too tight? Continue this process, stopping at your cheeks, your lower jaw, your neck, then your shoulders, until you've gone all the way down your body. If your mind drifts, bring it back to the body part you were focusing on.

→ LET TECH HELP

If you're having trouble incorporating mindfulness in your life, try downloading an app. Many allow you to set reminders on your phone to meditate at different

points in the day, and some even text you daily doses of inspiration. (Just remember to turn your phone off once you start meditating, since you don't want to be distracted by pings.) A few good ones to try:

Headspace teaches the ABCs of meditation; plus, you can also get mindfulness advice from former monk Andy Puddicombe. *headspace.com*

Calm offers guided meditations and "sleep stories" to help you get a good night's rest. *calm.com*

Coach helps you form a new habit and offers one-on-one consultations with a variety of mindfulness coaches. *coach.me*

Smiling Mind is a web- and app-based program developed by an Australian nonprofit. Its meditation and mindfulness exercises were designed by psychologists and educators to help bring balance to your life. *smilingmind.com.au*

Stop, Breathe & Think is designed to help users cope with conditions like stress, anxiety, depression and insomnia. It offers meditation instruction, along with 27 free meditation audios (more are available through a subscription). *stopbreathethink.org*

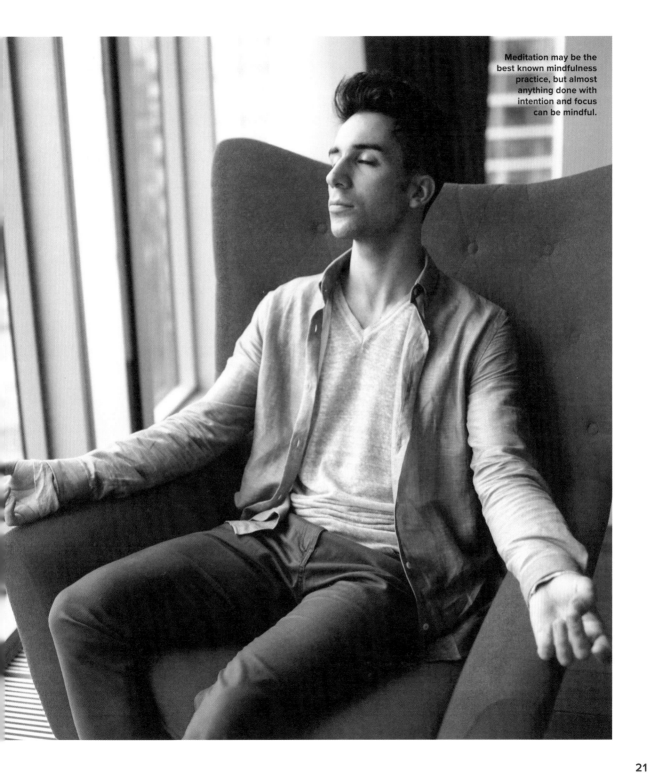

Meditation may be the best known mindfulness practice, but almost anything done with intention and focus can be mindful.

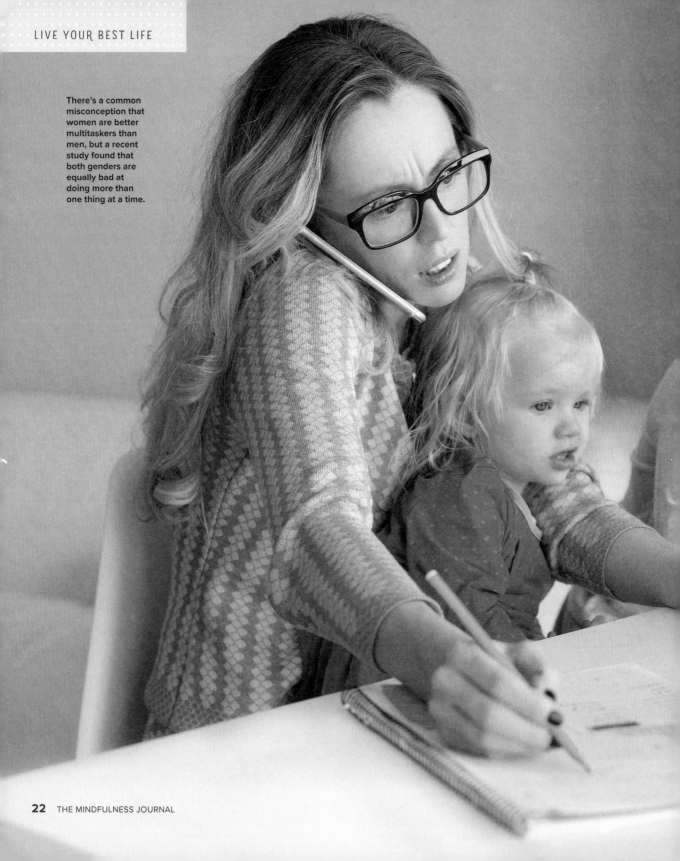

There's a common misconception that women are better multitaskers than men, but a recent study found that both genders are equally bad at doing more than one thing at a time.

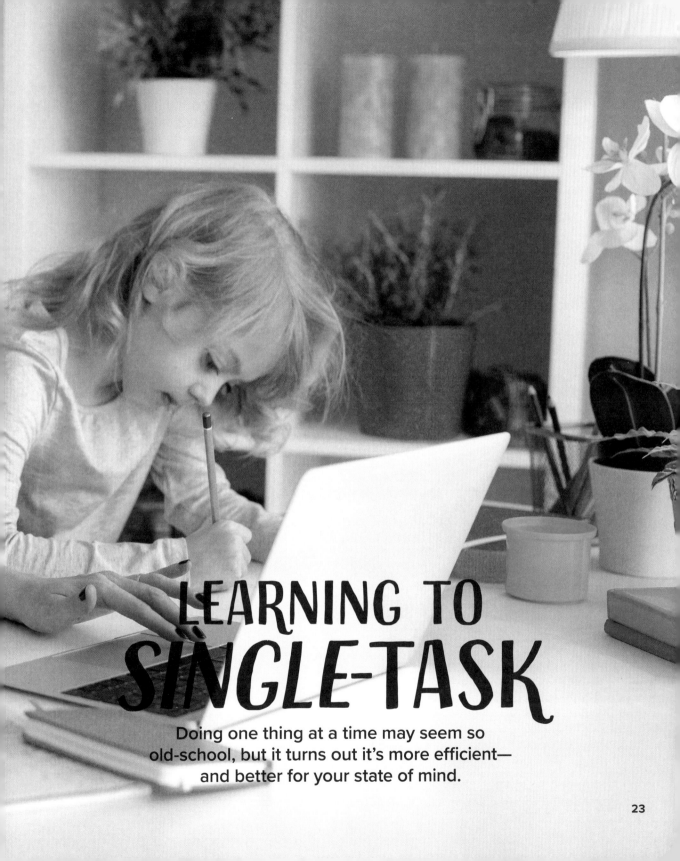

LEARNING TO SINGLE-TASK

Doing one thing at a time may seem so
old-school, but it turns out it's more efficient—
and better for your state of mind.

When you're simultaneously checking emails, shouting to Alexa to text your sister and ordering your kids' sports equipment, while fretting about an upcoming work presentation as you throw string cheese into school lunch bags, you may feel like you're getting so much more done.

But the reality is that multitasking only offers the *illusion* of productivity. Often, this is when stress levels are ramped up and more mistakes are made—which usually ends up taking more time in the long run.

REDEFINING THE JUGGLE

● The clinical (and, let's be honest, more accurate) term for doing more than one thing at a time is not multitasking but "task-switching," because in reality, you can't concentrate on more than one thing at a time. In fact, the American Psychological Association has calculated that all of the task-switching we do and all of the distractions caused by technology can cost a whopping 40 percent of someone's productive time.

But by learning to prioritize tasks, minimize distractions and focus on one thing at a time, you can actually do a better, more thorough job—and, #bonuspoints, feel calmer at the end of the day.

Mindfulness, which is the ability to fully focus on one thing at a time and be present in the moment, is the opposite of distractedly multitasking—and can be the key to solving it. "I believe it's the key to a healthier relationship with technology," says Christina Malecka, a Seattle-based psychotherapist and the founder of Digital Mindfulness Retreats.

A 2016 Case Western Reserve University meta-analysis of previous studies noted that it's estimated that the human mind wanders for roughly half of our waking hours, but that mindfulness has been shown to improve three qualities of attention—stability, control and efficiency.

Practices like meditation, yoga, tai chi or journaling "provide a foundation that makes it easier to step back, see the big picture, respond rather than react, and focus on one thing at a time," Malecka explains. This can help you in every aspect of your life, from home to office. Being mindful can also help

you refocus when your day starts to overwhelm you... and we've all had those days.

Ready to toss those multitasking habits to the curb? Consider trying some of these other actions to increase your focus.

MAKE A MASTER LIST

● There's the to-do list in your phone, the one on your at-home calendar, plus several Post-its scattered around the house. "It's impossible to start prioritizing if you don't really know all of the things you need to get done," notes Malecka. Gather them all, and be sure to include all of those things that swirl in your head and create a knot in your stomach. Many people find this list-making incredibly satisfying and can even help to reduce feelings of stress and anxiety.

LEARN TO PRIORITIZE

● Be honest, is No. 5 on your list really that important? And is No. 1 truly urgent? If it's hard for you to figure out, try using the task-prioritization method called the Eisenhower Matrix, which helps you prioritize tasks by assessing their level of importance, and deciding if they can be delegated or even taken off the list entirely (see illustration, below). Then assess what

The Eisenhower Matrix

Do First	**Do Later**
These are urgent things that need to be done ASAP.	These can be postponed, but do schedule a time to do them.
Delegate	**Eliminate**
It makes more sense to find someone else to do these.	These aren't important and can be crossed off your list.

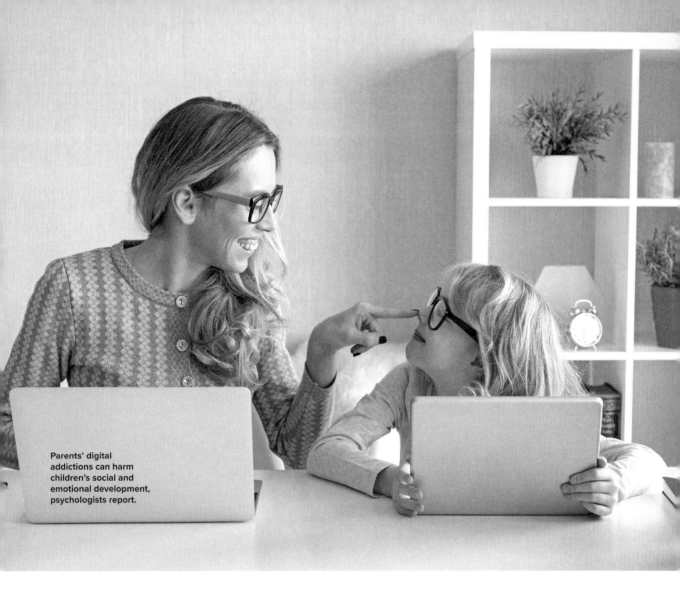

Parents' digital addictions can harm children's social and emotional development, psychologists report.

needs to be done today, and back-burner everything else that you can.

SET ASIDE CONCENTRATED BLOCKS OF TIME TO FOCUS ON ONE TASK

● Shut off all unnecessary technology. Close the door. Put on noise-canceling headphones if you work in a busy office. Do whatever it takes to remove unhelpful distractions. You will find you get more accomplished, which will, in turn, reduce your anxiety and increase your feelings of self-satisfaction.

IMMERSE YOURSELF IN NATURE

● Spending time outdoors is an ideal way to help you relax and open your mind to creative thoughts, and yet many of us suffer from what experts have labeled "nature deficit disorder." "Nature has the power to transform and awaken us," says Mark Coleman, a meditation teacher in Marin Country, California, and author of *Awake in the Wild: Mindfulness in Nature as a Path of Self Discovery.* "Yet in our busy, high-tech lives, we have lost the ability, sensitivity and skill to listen, feel and sense the natural world."

TAKING A DIGITAL DETOX

Stepping away from your screens will benefit your mindset, your quality of life and your relationships.

Do your devices have a death grip on your attention? Christina Malecka, a mental health counselor, has these suggestions for taking a break from technology:

→ **TURN OFF ALERTS AND PUSH NOTIFICATIONS**—and then set a time when you'll catch up with emails, texts and your social media accounts. (If you're worried about being out of touch, you can adjust your settings so you're only reachable by family members or other essential people.)

→ **PUT YOUR PHONE AWAY** when you are having social time with family or friends so that they know they are a priority. In a recent study from the City University of New York, researchers found that children expressed more distress when their mothers were using their cellphones, and that "mobile device use can have a negative impact on infant social-emotional functioning and parent-child interactions." "The No. 1 complaint I hear from children in my private counseling practice is that their mothers are always looking at their phones and not them," says Malecka. Leave your phone out of your physical reach during downtime. You're less likely to obsessively check it if you have to go to another room to get it.

→ **MAKE YOUR BEDROOM A TECH-FREE ZONE.** I know, I know, the thought of not watching Netflix in bed, on your iPad, is enough to cause a panic attack. Set a technology stop time every evening and stick to it—you *really* don't need to know that someone else liked your breakfast pic on Facebook before you go to sleep.

→ **HAVE EXPERIENCES WITHOUT DOCUMENTING THEM ON SOCIAL MEDIA.** You tend to take yourself out of the experience when you're more focused on just posting it to Instagram or Facebook.

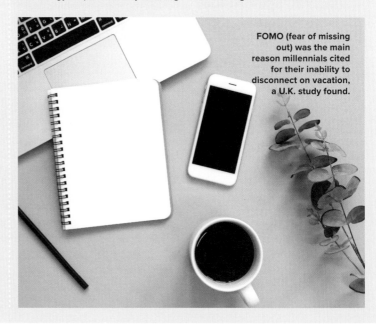

FOMO (fear of missing out) was the main reason millennials cited for their inability to disconnect on vacation, a U.K. study found.

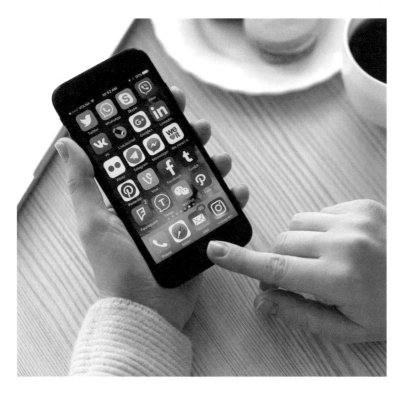

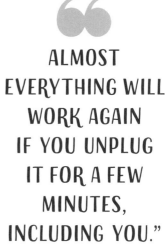

ALMOST EVERYTHING WILL WORK AGAIN IF YOU UNPLUG IT FOR A FEW MINUTES, INCLUDING YOU."

ANNE LAMOTT, NOVELIST

Studies have shown that time spent in nature significantly lowers blood pressure and dramatically increases a sense of well-being. So go out and watch the clouds. Feel the breeze. Count how many bird songs you hear. Just 10 minutes a day losing yourself in nature can make a difference.

SET ASIDE SOME UNSCHEDULED TIME IN YOUR DAY

● This will give your brain time to settle down and reboot. Take a walk by yourself, listen to music or just stare into space for a while, but do not look at your phone or fill in the silence with chatter.

RESIST THE CLICKBAIT

● If you're randomly clicking on whatever comes up on your screen, then you are letting Big Tech waste your time. Do you really need another sports bra, even one that promises to work miracles? Can you even afford the side table you just spent a good

20 minutes researching? Is Taylor Swift's latest Instagram post really that intriguing? Think before you click.

ONLY CHECK EMAILS AT SCHEDULED TIMES

● Instead of constantly interrupting your train of thought to answer emails and phone calls, set aside specific times to deal with them, when you will actually have time to give them your full attention.

PUT THE PRIORITY ON PEOPLE, NOT PHONES

● Another important reason we should shut out distractions is so we can have higher quality conversations and interpersonal relationships. "Digital and social media erodes real-time connection," notes Coleman. "Mindfulness enhances and deepens our capacity to have genuinely satisfying conversations and relationships."

REFRAMING NEGATIVE THOUGHT PATTERNS

"Think positive" might seem like the "it" mantra of our time, but experts say there's science behind the benefits of turning negative thinking to positive self-talk and optimism.

"Good morning, Pooh Bear,"
said Eeyore gloomily.
"If it is a good morning,"
he said. "Which I doubt."

Eyore, the perpetually gloomy gray donkey in the Winnie-the-Pooh books, is a classic poster child for negativity—depressed, morose and often pessimistic, a constant downer.

But are negative thought patterns a problem? It's really just being realistic about life, right?

Actually, our self-talk, positive or negative, impacts not only our perceptions of the world, but also the overall quality of our life. "How we talk to ourselves affects how we see ourselves and others, how we eat, love and experience life," says Cynthia Kane, certified meditation and mindfulness instructor, founder of The Intentional Communication Institute, and author of *How To Communicate Like a Buddhist*. "If you're constantly telling yourself that you can't do anything right, then nothing you do will be good enough. You could be praised for a job well done and not believe it. You could be given the opportunity to advance in your career and not accept it. You could get into a discussion with your partner and instead of listening,

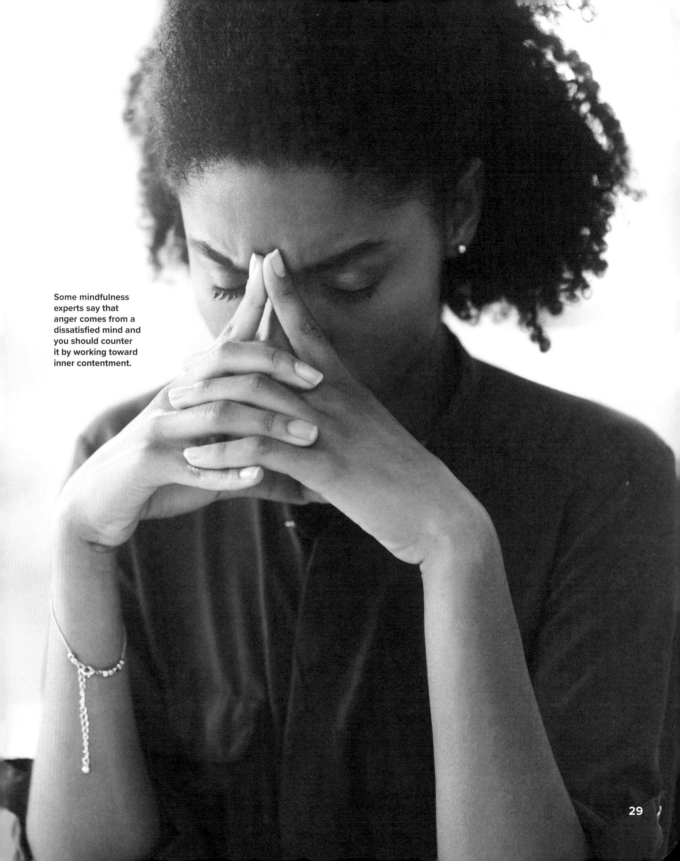

Some mindfulness experts say that anger comes from a dissatisfied mind and you should counter it by working toward inner contentment.

throw your hands up and announce, 'Well, I can't do anything right, can I?'"

These negative perceptions also directly affect our mood and interactions, because we anticipate poor outcomes, situations and relationships. In other words, how can you have a happy, peaceful, gratitude-filled life if you're not feeding and cultivating the same on the inside?

PROMOTING YOUR OWN SUFFERING

● According to Kane, negativity is always coupled with a judgment or a criticism. "Any time you say something that makes you feel sad, uncomfortable, 'less-than' in any way is negative self-talk," she says. "Language that promotes your own suffering is negative self-talk."

The good news is that not all negative thoughts are bad, especially when you're self-aware and learn to use them to redirect your behavior. "You shouldn't fear the negative, as you have to experience opposites—negative versus positive—to know what balance feels like for you," Kane says. "The negative can be seen and used as a poison, or it can be used as medicine, showing you where to pay more attention and heal, and where to allow more compassion, kindness and clarity." Simply reframing your perspective can shift your experience, mood and behavior.

AN INSTANTANEOUS EFFECT

● Thinking differently can truly happen in an instant, simply by paying attention to the words you use and thoughts you have. When you listen and identify your negative thought patterns, you can reframe your thinking and move toward speaking and acting more compassionately about yourself. "Exploring where the negative self-talk comes from (your past experiences, societal influences, etc.), and asking yourself questions—What judgment am I making? What do I know to be true?—creates space and distance from the negative self-talk," says Kane.

"It's breaking your attachment to it. Then you can release the old judgment through self-forgiveness or saying in the moment to yourself, 'This is negative self-talk and I choose to release it,'

so you can then move on to practicing balance." Once you do this, something interesting happens: You get a more honest perspective of yourself, rather than all of the false stories, negative opinions and harsh self-judgments that you've been constantly telling yourself.

THE POWER OF GRATITUDE

● Reframing isn't just about shifting and rebalancing, it's also about replacing negative thoughts with positive. For example, studies have shown that gratitude helps displace unhealthy moods, attitudes and experiences with a sense of appreciation and good fortune. "We see ourselves and our lives differently when we look at them through the lens of gratitude and appreciation," Kane says. "This can be a quick fix to help shift us out of negative self-talk; however, it doesn't get to the root of it."

That said, finding a new mantra, a happy-statement T-shirt or a coffee mug with an uplifting quote isn't necessarily the answer if you're just replacing negative self-talk with positive affirmations that aren't true. "Doing so would simply be going to the other extreme," Kane says. The trick is finding what's positive about a negative situation, which is more balanced and truthful, she adds.

POSITIVITY PAYOFFS

● Studies show that optimism isn't just good for your well-being, but leads to better finances, stronger relationships and the desire to make a positive impact in the world, too. "Most people want to be optimistic and see themselves this way, but when it comes to their own self-image and self-communication, it's more a belief than a reality," Kane says. "Part of the practice of achieving balanced communication with yourself is to include optimism in your thinking and self-talk, but only to the extent that it is true for you."

EVALUATING YOUR INNER CRITIC

● So how do you know whether your negative self-talk qualifies as balanced, or a tad too negative? Your inner critic doesn't have to be cruel or relentless in order to impact you negatively. Kane describes it as any time you're not speaking to yourself with honesty, compassion and kindness. "To speak to yourself [positively] means you respect and care for yourself, believe that who you are, as you are, is enough," she says. "That you have all you need within you to be able to take care of yourself and live well. To incorporate this way of speaking into your day-to-day is a practice of being comfortable with who you are—and the best way to become friendly toward yourself is through a meditation practice."

A LONG-TERM REMEDY

● Meditation not only helps you shift out of a negative spiral, but it also helps you prevent or sidestep situations where you might normally be overwhelmed by, or engage in, negative self-talk. We all have negative thoughts, but once you start paying attention to them while meditating, you'll notice their frequency and the toll they take on your mood and outlook. That's how you'll know when you need to reframe them. As Kane says, "You can allow negative thoughts to be there; they aren't the enemy. But when you become absorbed in them, and they're taking you away from what it is you want to be focusing on or distracting you from doing what you want to be doing or living the way you want to be living, then it's helpful to practice shifting out of them."

That's because meditating trains your brain to concentrate on one thing at a time, to be in the moment and respond thoughtfully and consciously, instead of reacting emotionally to situations.

Once you learn to change how you think or act in response to negative thoughts, you can take charge of your life rather than be ruled by emotions, especially ones that are often not true or extreme. "It's about how you respond to the emotion you're feeling and learn to live alongside it instead of being led around by it. In the moment, this looks like noticing your anger or frustration or stress, acknowledging it, taking a breath, labeling it—I'm feeling anger, frustration— then putting it to the side and coming back to the

present moment to choose a different response," says Kane. "Ask yourself, how do I want to feel instead? Calm, relaxed? Then what does that look like? Maybe it looks like breathing, watching what's happening and not getting involved, excusing yourself from a situation."

Practicing this reframed response on a daily basis will help you become, if not exactly a carefree Tigger type, then at least less of an Eeyore.

THE SEVEN TYPES OF NEGATIVE SELF-TALK

Meditation and mindfulness instructor Cynthia Kane says these thoughts are untrue, unhelpful or unkind. When a thought comes up, evaluate it to see if it fits into one of these categories:

1 OVERREACTION
"Everything is terrible."

2 PERSONALIZATION
"Why is this happening to me?"

3 ABSOLUTE LANGUAGE
"I'm a bad person."

4 ASSUMPTION
"He thinks I'm not good enough."

5 EXPECTATION
"This isn't how it's supposed to be."

6 COMPARISON
"Why can't I be like her?"

7 REGRET
"If I hadn't done that..."

THE ART OF
LETTING GO

Instead of ruminating about the past or worrying about the future, try being present; it's essential to becoming more mindful.

When I was 12, I went away to sleepover camp near Yosemite National Park. I spent the months before I went worrying: What should I pack? Would I make any friends? Would I get homesick? Would I be eaten by bears? I spent the first few days of camp worrying: What if I hadn't packed the right clothes? Did the counselors like me? Would I ever learn all the words to the camp song? A few days in, we were told that we were to go off into the woods and find a place to sit for an hour and be alone. I found this task very...worrying.

As I sat there, I worried about peckish bears, about what the other campers were doing and about whether I would make it through the whole hour. But gradually I began to notice the birds singing away in the pine trees, the smell of the needles and the sounds of the breeze in the branches and the gurgling of a nearby brook. I looked up at the steep granite walls towering into the bright blue sky. I finally took in that I was in one of the most beautiful places in the whole wide world. A feeling of joy tingled through my body. The hour was over in what seemed like a flash.

When we all gathered again, we regaled each other with our discoveries. Our counselors told us that we had just experienced living in the moment, and that it was something we could do all the time, no matter where we were. They were right.

A TIMELESS MESSAGE

● This lesson that I learned from those counselors has been touted for years by everyone from the Buddha to Oprah, and more and more research is showing that the seemingly simple practice of being present has a myriad of health benefits and can lead to happier lives. "Science is catching up with spiritual teachings to invite all of us to have some kind of practice to bring

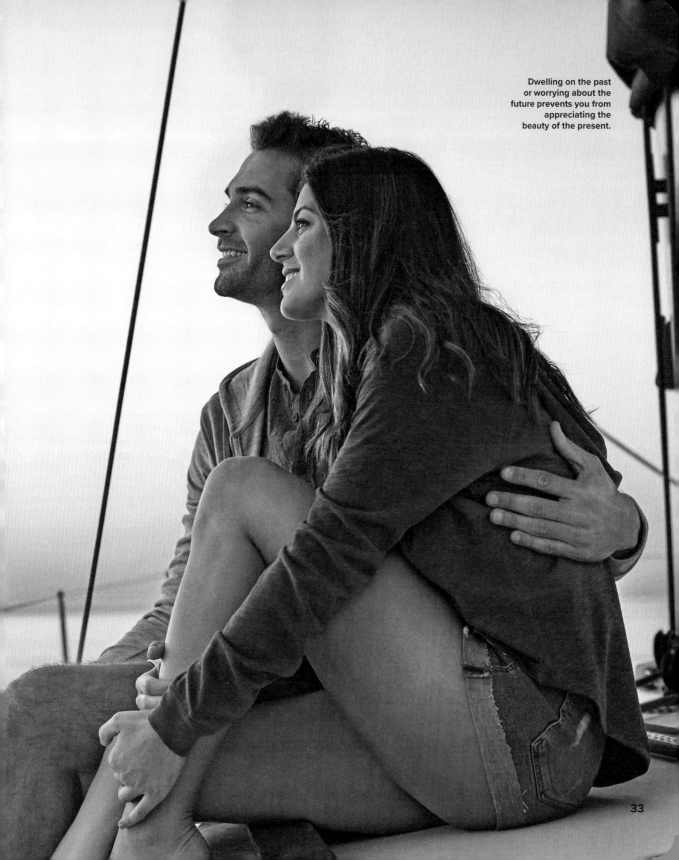

Dwelling on the past or worrying about the future prevents you from appreciating the beauty of the present.

33

us to the present," says Christa Santangelo, PhD, a clinical psychologist and assistant clinical professor at University of California, San Francisco, and author of *A New Theory of Teenagers: Seven Transformational Strategies to Empower You and Your Teen.*

But finding such a practice is easier said than done, particularly in the 21st century, with its hustle and bustle and pressure to go, go, go, and smartphones designed to distract us (see sidebar). Like 12-year-old me (and much-older me), we ruminate about the past and we fret about the future. When we do this, we are "skipping the present moment altogether," says Jesse Torgerson, a dynamic breathwork therapist in Los Angeles and New York City. She points out that we are sacrificing the reality of what is actually going on in the present moment for "our experience of a memory from the past or our imagination of what the future might hold. Thus, we are disconnected from our actual present moment experience and location, which is the source of anxiety for most people."

This fretting triggers the release of stress hormones, and if we continue to worry, we run the risk of chronic stress, which can lead to health problems including heart disease, trouble sleeping, fertility issues, indigestion, depression and forgetfulness.

The question is, then, exactly how do we live in the moment? "It is very achievable," says Santangelo. "Being in the present is in a certain way our natural state. When we're on vacation and we see a beautiful sunset, it's not difficult to engage in the moment. We can learn how to replicate these 'vacation moments' in our everyday lives."

"Consciously breathing is the most effective technique I know to enter into the present moment," says Torgerson. "Noticing the sensation of the inhale and the exhale brings a person into the experience of their body, their state of being and their actual present-moment location."

Experts say it can also be helpful to let your body settle into the moment, to feel yourself yielding to gravity. You can do a body scan and allow yourself to notice the sensations that come with that. Note what you hear, see, taste, smell and feel. Thoughts will come into your mind. Simply acknowledge them

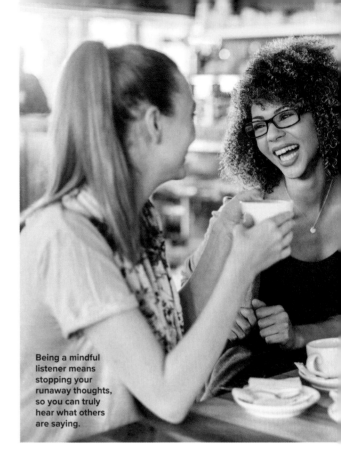

Being a mindful listener means stopping your runaway thoughts, so you can truly hear what others are saying.

and return to the sensations. Emotions will also arise. Santangelo notes the importance of accepting and allowing these. "It's OK to be sad or angry or uncomfortable or afraid, to allow the radical honesty of your emotions."

It's important to let go of any perfectionism or ideas of how this should feel, or should be done. Just be present with everything that comes up. Santangelo urges patience. "Many of my patients feel that they can't stay focused on the present moment, that it's too hard. But I remind them that we need to be gentle with ourselves. The Buddha apparently figured out how to do it, but it might take some of us a lot longer."

This acceptance and awareness can also be brought to daily tasks like washing dishes or eating. Try allowing yourself to slow down and feel the warmth of the water, the smoothness of the dishes. Savor each bite and don't distract yourself with screen-

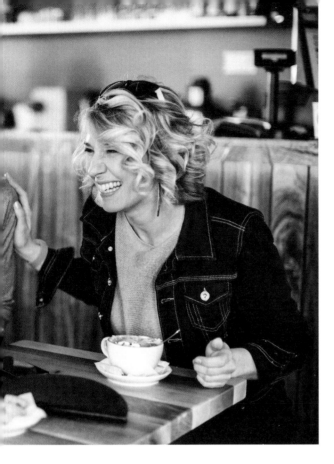

time. Keep this Zen proverb in mind: "When walking, walk; when eating, eat."

As I learned long ago in Yosemite, being aware of the present is a gift. "We each get such a short moment to experience the mystery, the struggle, and the miracle of life in a human form," *Eat, Pray, Love* author Elizabeth Gilbert recently wrote in an Instagram post. "Don't miss our brief moment to be alive.... Feel the air on your skin. Drink a glass of water. Touch the soft fur of an animal.... Cry, if you need to. But be here..."

As you do all of this you will find, as I did all those years ago in the woods, that you are better able to appreciate the beauty of the moment and to be present and available for your relationships and your work—for everything in your life. As Torgerson says, you will be more and more aware of the "well-being, safety and wholeness of the now."

—*Katherine Wessling*

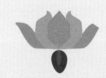

STOP THE DIGITAL CHATTER

Our smartphones are Public Enemy No. 1 when it comes to being in the moment. Their pings and dings yank us out of the now by getting us to pick them up and start scrolling. And texting. And so on.

Every time we switch to a new task (say, from writing a report to checking texts, then Instagram, then email...), there is a stop-start process that happens in our brain. This wastes time and can lead to mistakes. Plus, we are no longer in the present.

Here are a few ways to stop this digital interference with your blissful state of being in the now:

➔ Keep your phone in silent mode unless you are waiting for a truly important call.

➔ Turn off the "vibrate on silent" setting (vibrating is still distracting!).

➔ Turn off notifications (all of them—phone calls, social media, news alerts, texts, etc.).

➔ Hide your phone from view.

➔ Turn the color scheme to black and white (search for color filters and chose grayscale); it's less appealing.

➔ Create a screen saver that makes you think about being more in the moment. Disable touch ID (entering a passcode makes you think about what you're doing, and whether you need to do it).

➔ Set aside specific times to check your phone. Hell, even mindlessly surf the internet if you are so inclined! A good rule of thumb is mid-morning, late afternoon and no later than two hours before bed.

I WENT ON A
SILENT RETREAT

Could you go five days without talking? It sounds unpleasant, if not impossible—but one woman found that it was both liberating and transformative.

oving wordlessly through the cafeteria, I simultaneously notice the smells of curry and fried food. Plates ping and cutlery clinks as a line of strangers flow through the food lines filling their plates for the midday meal. Eerily absent is the sound of human voices.

Ever wish you could just turn off the noise? Well, here was my opportunity. This was the second day of a seven-day retreat and we had officially entered into the silent phase. I load my plate from the salad bar and slip into a seat across from a fellow participant.

Automatically, her head lifts, aware of my presence. She gives me a silent nod and then sinks back into experiencing her lunch. We share the energy of a common human connection and yet we have been relieved of having to introduce ourselves or make small talk. Liberated from this typical, and oftentimes frightening, type of social interaction, my energy focuses on savoring my meal with a peripheral awareness of the human motion swirling around. Cottage cheese never tasted this creamy and good, or perhaps I had just never noticed!

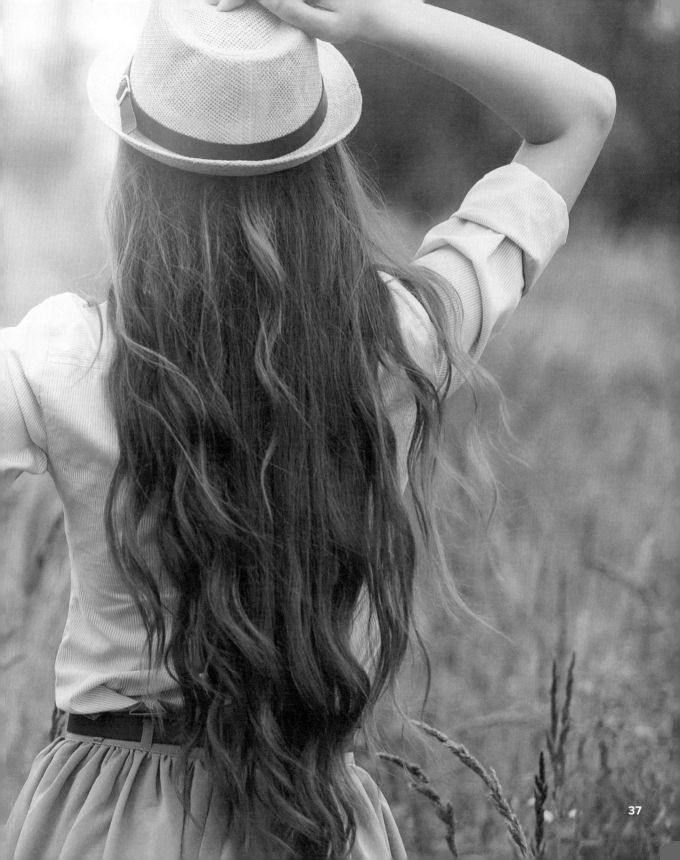

MINDFULNESS 101

A number of years ago, I was reading about the compassion meditation research conducted by neuroscientist Richard Davidson, PhD, at the University of Wisconsin's Center for Healthy Minds in Madison, where I lived at the time, and how it leads to greater happiness. I decided to attend the drop-in meditation practice called the Joy of Living (JOL) hosted by Tergar, a meditation community where Davidson occasionally facilitates the teachings, because, frankly, who doesn't want to become happier? Davidson, who's also a professor of psychology and psychiatry at the University of Wisconsin-Madison, calls meditation a "radical act of compassion."

This secular curriculum was developed by Yongey Mingyur Rinpoche, a Tibetan Buddhist meditation master, who makes these profound ancient practices both accessible and comical. Enamored by both the practice and the community, I signed up for a weeklong group JOL retreat at St. John's University in Collegeville, Minnesota.

Already intimidated by the prospect of meditating six to eight hours a day, my trepidation grew when I arrived on campus that Monday evening to find out that five of those days would be in silence! No noise, no "toys," including all manner of technological connectivity, and even intimacy (partners were encouraged to stay in separate rooms)! Reading was allowed as long as it supported practice.

Our first full day began with a focus on both attention and intention. The purpose of this silent retreat was to bring awareness to our own innate goodness by meditating on kindness and compassion for ourselves and others. The idea is that this will then ripple outward, bringing greater happiness to ourselves and those around us.

The schedule was intense. Morning meditation started at 7 a.m. with six half-hour sessions (with five-minute breaks in between), punctuated by an hour of teaching, a half-hour tea break in the middle, one or two half-hour walking meditations, and a final hour of meditation before lunch. The afternoon worked basically the same. After dinner, the evening ended with a group teaching.

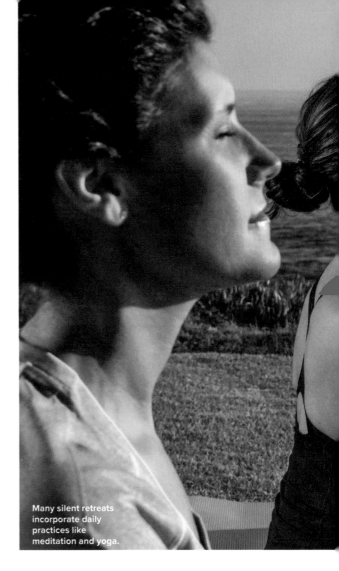

Many silent retreats incorporate daily practices like meditation and yoga.

As we continued this pattern throughout the week, I sensed a heightened awareness to sounds, like the wind or the birds outside my window. I paid more attention to taste, movement and how my body was feeling, all with a greater sense of wonder and appreciation. The environment for this exploration felt safe and supportive. Guided by our teachers and the warm energy of others, I began to feel my heart and mind open. This can lead to what Mingyur Rinpoche calls the "waterfall effect," whereby thoughts and emotions flow freely, bringing forth all manner of "debris," which can sometimes be

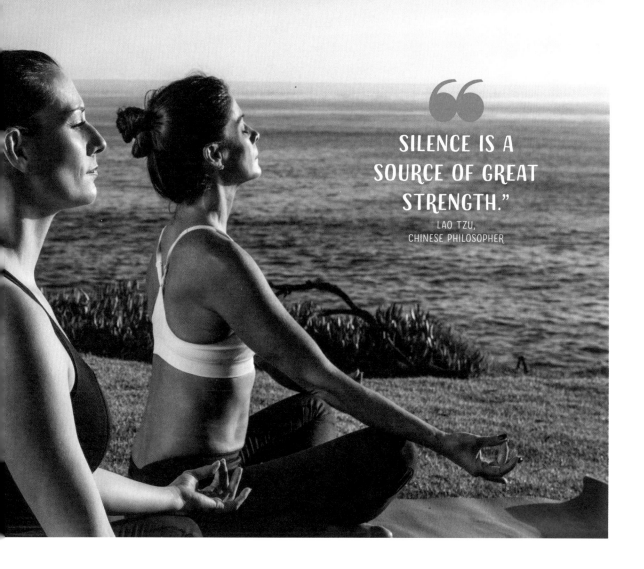

> ## SILENCE IS A SOURCE OF GREAT STRENGTH."
>
> LAO TZU,
> CHINESE PHILOSOPHER

overwhelming. It was not uncommon to see people in tears, including myself. But we reached out to each other, in the process developing a powerful sense of compassion and connection. My awareness, feeling of connection and clarity of perspective all increased in ways I can only describe as transformative.

It has been said that life is beguiling and the mind is fickle. We spend much of our time in busy work, running from activity to activity, juggling demanding requirements and emotional tugs, whether real or perceived. There is rarely an opportunity to inquire within without distraction or verbal interaction. One thing I realized was that it's not so scary in there. And when we become intimate with our fears and anxieties, in a sense befriending them rather than pushing them away, they seem to dissipate. This self-compassion then begins to ripple out to others.

On the last day of the retreat, the cafeteria begins to hum with joyful talk, as conversation is again allowed. Happy, yet hesitant to be released from our silence, stories and insights were shared. It felt as though a weight had been lifted and the path forward was a little clearer.

—*Sandra Fernandez*

THE THANK-YOU PROJECT

Making gratitude a habit is one of the most powerful ways to enhance your physical and emotional well-being. Here's how to get started.

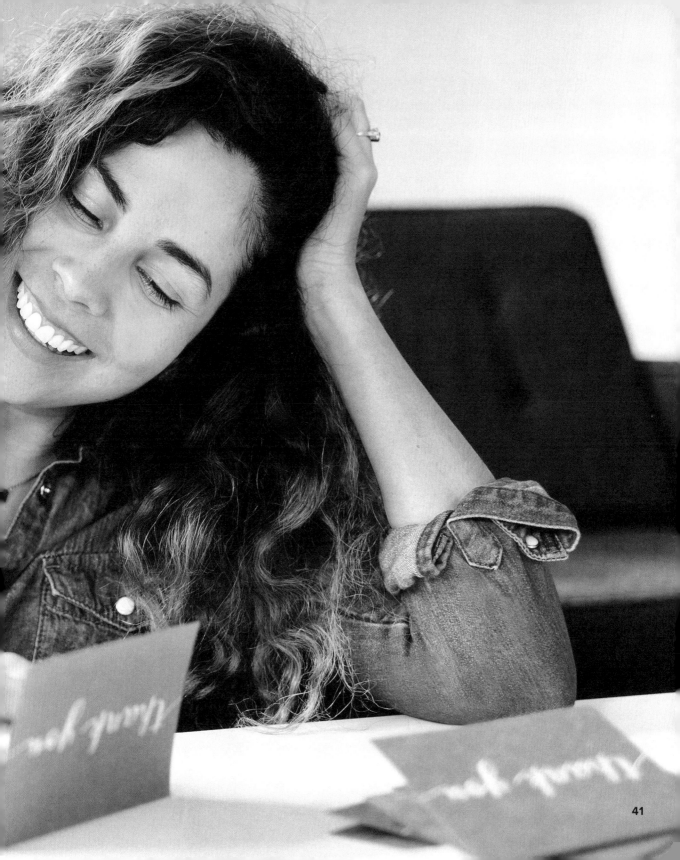

If you're like most Americans, there's a good chance that most years, you've sat around the Thanksgiving table with your family as each person takes a requisite turn expressing their thank-yous. Maybe it was for something trivial like the delicious meal that Mom prepared, or perhaps you gushed about the beautiful new baby you recently welcomed into your family. Either way, you probably felt all warm and cozy on the inside as you dug into that slice of pumpkin pie.

If giving thanks feels so good, why don't we do it more often? Well, like anything else worth our while, thinking in terms of gratitude is a learned skill. "Our brain is more likely to shift to the negative, in an attempt to protect us and safeguard us," says Anne Deidre, the bestselling author of *Intuition: 7 Basic Instincts to Change Your Life*. "Going into the realm of gratitude takes getting used to. It's about forming a habit so it becomes an automated practice."

Although shifting your mindset to one of gratitude takes a little practice, the good news is that the payoff is powerful. Taking the time to count your blessings, both big and small, can greatly benefit your overall well-being, from helping to mitigate depression, stress and anxiety, to making you feel happier in your relationships and throughout your daily life.

In fact, a 2017 study in *The Review of Communication* reported that the more subjects expressed gratitude, the more long-term success they experienced in their relationships. Similarly, research out of the University of Georgia found that couples who were vocal about their appreciation for one another had a stronger marital bond.

What's more, in 2019 researchers found that thankfulness helped improve the quality of life for those dealing with a life-threatening illness. And a 2014 study found that more-grateful individuals were better at coping with trauma and high-stress situations.

Deidre, who's also a speaker and an intuitive life coach, believes that being more appreciative can also help our bodies feel better. "I find that thoughts lead to emotions, and emotions lead to the physical," she says. "By practicing gratitude, you're making room for more joy." Another bonus: Doing so will also help enhance your intuition, she adds, so you can make better (and less stressful) decisions, no matter the size.

Bottom line: "When you get into a continuous habit of having your go-to be gratitude, you're not going to be up and down as much on that emotional roller coaster," Deidre adds. "You're evening out your life streams, your flow."

Want to get started? Read on for some simple ways to make thankfulness as second nature as brushing your teeth...or asking for that second slice of pie.

WRITE IT DOWN
● "When Oprah Winfrey came out with her gratitude journal," Deidre recalls, "it certainly started a conversation." Writing down the things you're grateful for on a daily basis creates awareness for all the good in your life, whether that's your dinner, the book that you're reading or your relationship, she says. "There's something that happens when you put pen to paper—the expression of it. You're noticing things, giving them credibility, and that helps you to expand."

TRY IT Deidre recommends jotting down your list in the evening (a simple drugstore notebook will do). "It's a good time to review the day," she says. "I find that going into that space of gratitude before bed promotes better sleep." Science backs her up: A 2009 study in the *Journal of Psychosomatic Research* found that gratitude helped people sleep more soundly and for a longer duration.

Prefer to do things in the a.m.? That works, too, Deidre says. "The key is to fit it into *your* day, in order to make it a habit."

BE A GRATITUDE DETECTIVE
● On those days when you're feeling less than grateful, when you feel like you're trekking through mud (hey, we've all been there), it's time to dig deeper, Deidre advises. "Even if you don't feel like

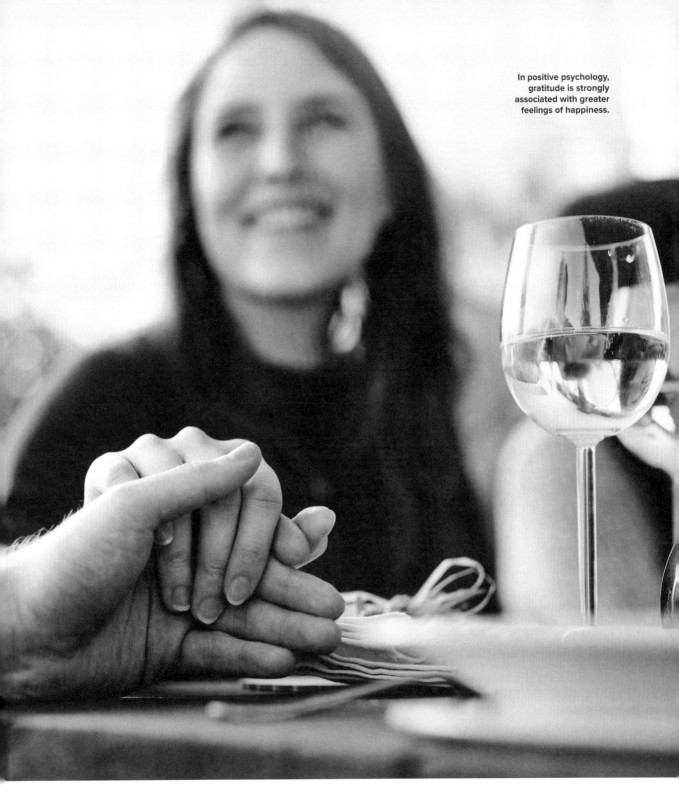

In positive psychology, gratitude is strongly associated with greater feelings of happiness.

A gratitude jar helps remind us of all the big *and* small things there are to appreciate in our lives.

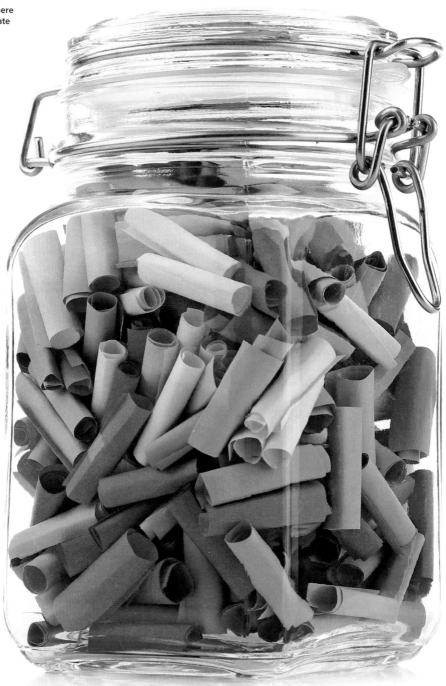

there is a blessing in a particular situation or day, be open to discovery. When you establish a consistent practice of shifting thoughts, there are fewer and fewer of those emotional upheavals."

TRY IT Understand that there is meaning behind everything, and try to pinpoint the positive in the situation at hand, Deidre suggests, even if your overall feelings tend to be negative.

SET AN INTENTION

● "The thing about intentions is, sometimes we're so used to being enmeshed in a certain mental pattern," Deidre says. "To get yourself out of that, you need to do something different." So when you wake up in the morning, make a point to establish a gratitude goal for the day, which also helps bring you back to the present. You can even try writing it down or selecting it as your screen saver on your phone.

TRY IT Your daily intention can be something as simple as, "I intend to feel grateful today" or "I'm grateful for the moments of joy I'm going to experience today." And there's a good chance that doing so will translate into better self-care during the day, according to research in the journal *Personality and Individual Differences*, which reported that people who felt thankful on the regular were more likely to engage in activities that benefit well-being, such as exercising and visiting the doctor.

PAY IT FORWARD

● Dedicating some of your time and energy to service has a sneaky way of making you appreciate all that you have. Numerous studies have found that volunteering boosts overall life satisfaction, happiness and wellness. And the more joyful and healthier we are, the more likely we are to navigate from a place of gratitude.

TRY IT Don't know where to begin? Resources like volunteermatch.org and createthegood.org can help you find volunteering opportunities in your city or your neighborhood.

LET IT SIMMER

● "Consciously linking moments with gratitude brings more awareness and mindfulness to each moment," Deidre says. "When you notice something you feel grateful for, have a practice of really feeling it in your heart," she recommends.

TRY IT When you catch yourself feeling thankful, hold onto that feeling for as long as possible. And when something annoying happens, recall to mind the things you truly appreciate in your life, which will help you put life's setbacks and disappointments in perspective.

TRY THE "NO COMPLAINTS" CHALLENGE

● Whether you're conscious of it or not, there's a good chance you're guilty of complaining—otherwise known as recounting a story to another in a negative way. And since grumbling is pretty much anti-gratitude, the idea behind a zero-complaints-allowed challenge is to increase your awareness with the goal of minimizing your kvetching.

TRY IT Make a "vow" to not complain about a thing for a designated period of time—say 24 hours or the eight hours you spend at work (or even a full month if you're feeling ambitious). You can do it!

A WAY OF LIFE

● Creating a gratitude jar and filling it with slips of paper listing moments and things you're grateful for allows you to reflect on all the positive things in your life. Sure, you could just read your journal, but there's something more fun—and visceral—about reading a jar-full of your notes.

TRY IT Place a mason jar (or any container)—along with a small pad of paper or Post-its and a pen—in a designated spot, such as on your nightstand or near your keys. Every day, make it a point to jot down one thing you're grateful for, fold it up and put it in the jar. Then, at the end of the month, read all your notes in one sitting.

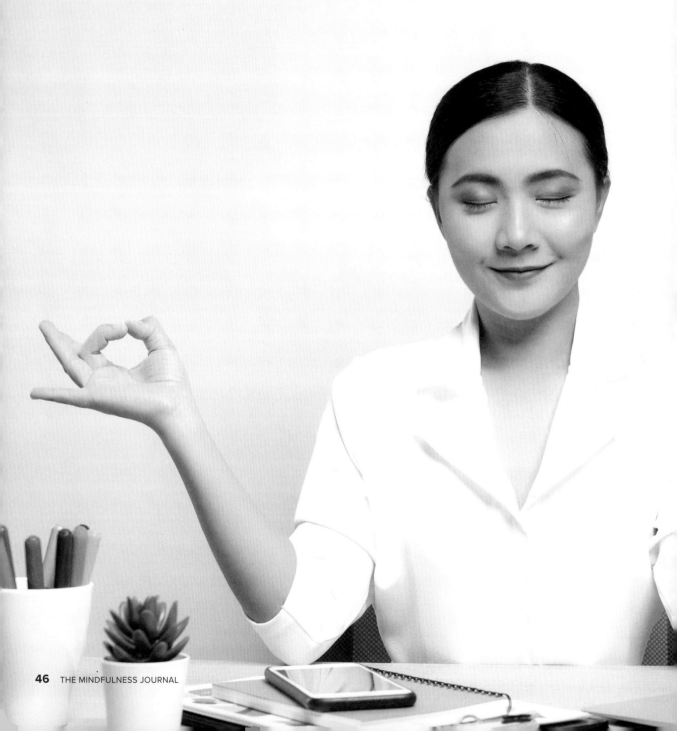

CAN WORK BE MORE ZEN?

No one will ever mistake it
for a Buddhist monastery, but you
can make your office more
conducive to a mindful lifestyle.

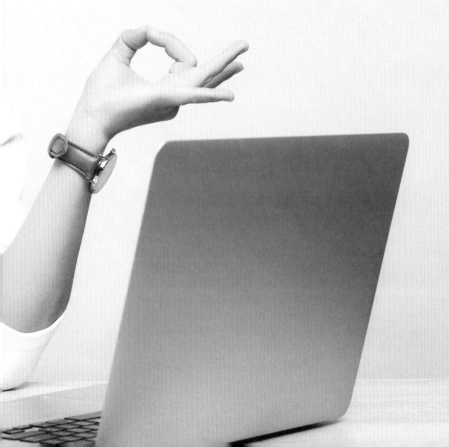

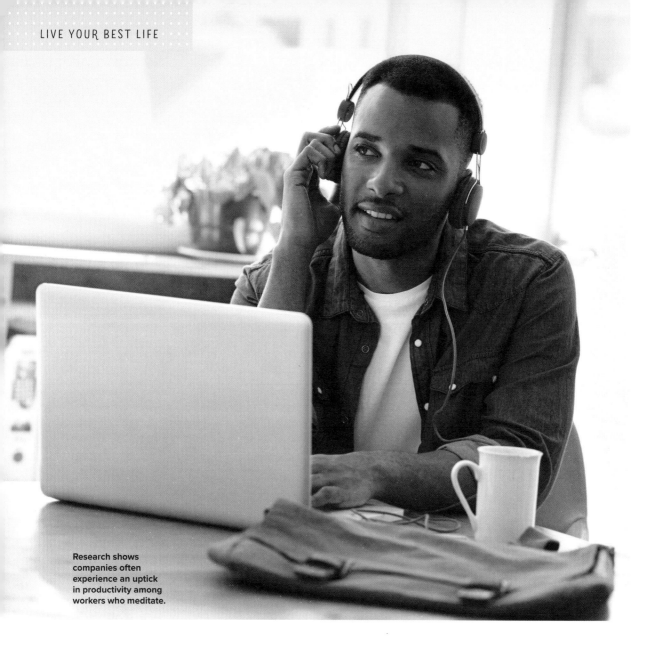

Research shows companies often experience an uptick in productivity among workers who meditate.

We spend a huge chunk of our time at work, but open office spaces, endless digital notifications, the disappearance of the lunch break, and after-hours emails make working 9 to 5 more like working 24/7. "It's important to apply some of the principles of mindfulness to your work life, so you don't burn out and instead remain as productive as possible," says

Julie Morgenstern, a productivity and organizational consultant in New York and author of *Organizing From the Inside Out.* "If you look at the people who perform the best at work, you'll notice one thing in common, whether they're the CEO or the CEO's assistant: They incorporate mindfulness techniques into their everyday routines." Consider trying some of these expert-approved strategies:

CREATE MINDFUL TRANSITIONS

• "Make sure that you're not carrying anything across your home or office threshold from the other part of your life that will dilute your presence wherever you are," says Morgenstern. On your way out of the office, for example, focus on the feeling of wind on your face rather than ruminating on what your boss said in your last meeting. Driving home, notice the strange shapes of clouds or the sounds of birds, rather than thinking about your kids' crazy after-school schedules. "This is also a good time to set intentions—ask yourself what you want to communicate to your kids when you get home, which is most likely that you love them, instead of screaming at them to do their homework while you're frantically checking texts on your phone," says Morgenstern. By focusing on being present at work, and then being present at home, you'll maximize efficiency and reap the best of both words.

TAKE MINI-BREATHING BREAKS AT WORK

• Even five minutes of relaxation will allow you to recharge your mental batteries, says Milana Perepyolkina, a wellness expert in Salt Lake City and author of *Dark Chocolate for the Soul*. Periodically throughout the day, while sitting at your desk, sit quietly with your eyes closed and breathe slowly and deeply for a few minutes. Inhale and hold your breath for a few seconds, exhale and hold your breath again. Try to focus solely on your breathing, with no other thoughts running through your head.

TUNE IN

• People who listen to music at work complete tasks more quickly and are more creative than those who don't, according to a study published in *Psychology of Music*. "Music allows you to still be physically present while emotionally in another space," explains Lauren Cook, MMFT, a therapist at the University of San Diego's student counseling center. Try listening to baroque music, like Vivaldi's *The Four Seasons*, which University of Maryland researchers found improved mood and boosted concentration at work.

FROM CUBICLE TO YOUR CALM PLACE

Whether you have a corner office or are stuck in the middle of a busy open space, you'll want to make your work area as peaceful and relaxing as possible. Here's how.

→ BRING IN A PLANT OR TWO
Even seeing just a little green can do wonders for your mindset. A 2015 study published in the *Journal of Physiological Anthropology* found that young adults exposed to indoor plants reported feeling calmer and had lower blood pressure.

→ INVEST IN A DIFFUSER
Having a calming smell, like lavender, or a refreshing one, like peppermint or lemon, in your work space is a great way to help support a more zen and focused environment, says Jessica Bird Hagestedt, a functional wellness coach based in San Diego.

→ SELECT COLORS STRATEGICALLY
Soft blues and greens are soothing, while yellows and oranges are stimulating. Vibrant blues, greens and light purples will help give you energy and keep you calm as you carry on, says Jesal Trivedi, CEO and founder of Aduri, a meditation-cushion company.

→ START A DAILY GRATITUDE PRACTICE
Hang a whiteboard that lets you acknowledge the things in your life that you are appreciative of, suggests mindfulness consultant DeAnn Wandler-Vukovich. Or just keep a running list in a journal somewhere on your desk.

PRACTICE SOME SELF-CARE

● It's easy to get overwhelmed with deadlines or new tasks, but visualization can be a powerful aid in relaxing muscles that often become tight or tense with added stress, says Tiffany Ryan, PhD, MSW, LMT, RYT, director of the Complex Trauma Research Institute in Portland, Oregon, and founder of massage company Yomassage. She recommends putting a small ball (like a tennis ball) under your feet (or putting one on your low back while sitting in a chair), then closing your eyes and visualizing your muscles melting over the ball. Also build in a couple of stretching breaks during the day. "Stretching activates the same sensory receptors as massage and can also act as a stress reducer," explains Ryan. One good move: Fold forward by bending at the waist, letting your arms hang and moving an ear toward the shoulder on each side to release stress in your neck.

EAT LUNCH MINDFULLY

● It's easy to fall into a pattern of gobbling down a sandwich while you're also banging away at your computer, but you'll benefit from spending as little as 10 to 15 minutes away from your desk, says DeAnn Wandler-Vukovich, a mindfulness educational and workplace consultant in the Washington, D.C. metro area. It's also important to savor your meal without distractions, eating slowly and engaging your senses so that you enjoy its flavor, texture and smell. Besides refueling with healthy, brain-powering foods (think fish, blueberries, raw carrots, avocados, nuts, seeds and small squares of chocolate), keep yourself hydrated with fruit-infused water throughout the day. "Don't just guzzle the water down—sip it with the same mindful awareness that you gave to your lunch," she advises.

STAY OFF EMAIL AFTER HOURS

● Yes, occasionally you need to bring work home, but try to avoid checking your email after hours as much as possible. Just the anticipation of having to respond to work emails at home causes stress, according to a 2018 Virginia Tech study. If that's not an option, establish boundaries by letting your boss know your off-hour email windows or providing a schedule of when you'll be able to respond. It's also a good idea to avoid emails as well as all forms of social media for at least the first and last hour of your day, advises Morgenstern. "By resisting these edges, you retrain yourself that your world will not fall apart if you're not checking all your accounts 24/7," she says. "It helps you stay focused and present in the moment."

STRUCTURE YOUR OFF-WORK TIME

● "People need structure, but most of us put that into our work—we don't know how to handle our weekends and they fall through our fingers," explains Morgenstern. Her advice: Think of your weekend as separated into seven blocks of time: Friday evening, Saturday morning, afternoon and evening, and Sunday morning, afternoon and evening. "Assign different things to those blocks —for example, tell yourself that Friday night is your time to relax and recharge by eating takeout and watching a funny movie," she says. Include things like exercise, self-care, seeing friends and spending family time together.

GET QUALITY Z'S

● Sleeping less than six hours each night is one of the best predictors of on-the-job burnout, according to the National Sleep Foundation. There's good reason for that: Sleep helps keep you mindful at the office by allowing you to recover from distractions faster and improving your ability to make split-second decisions. You can slip into dreamland more quickly with a before-bed meditation: People who do so report less insomnia, fatigue and depression, according to a 2015 study in *JAMA Internal Medicine*. Morgenstern recommends choosing a calming focus, such as a sound like "om" or a positive word like "relax" or "peace" and repeating it, either aloud or silently, as you inhale or exhale. When you notice your mind wandering, simply take another deep breath and return to focus on the mantra you've chosen.

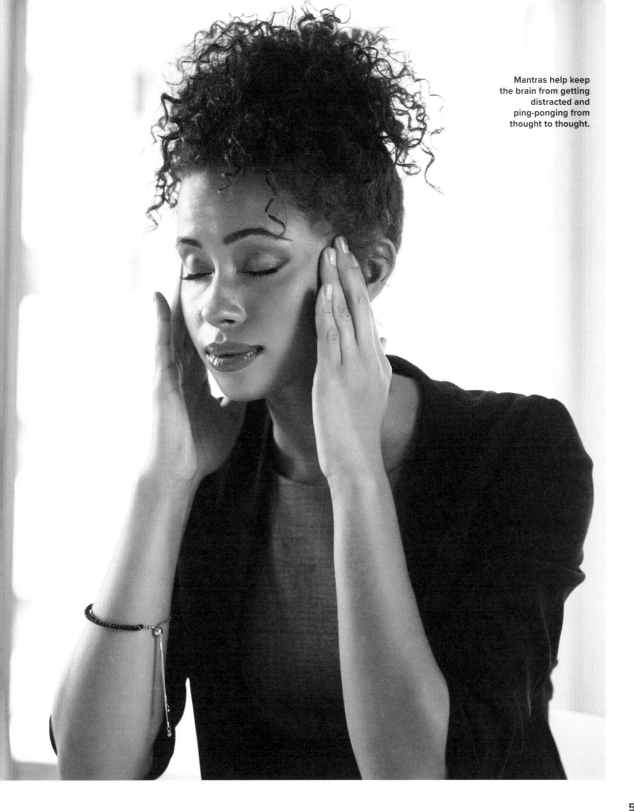

Mantras help keep the brain from getting distracted and ping-ponging from thought to thought.

THE BENEFITS OF DECLUTTERING

Making room for *just* what really matters brings balance back into your life.

Is clutter stressing you out? If so, you aren't alone. (And you don't have to be a candidate for *Hoarders* to be affected by it.) In a world where we can order whatever we want with the click of a mouse, many of us are drowning in "stuff," and we also seem to have less and less time to deal with it all. So it's no surprise that clutter, and the distraction and anxiety it can cause, is a problem for so many of us—even when we don't always realize it.

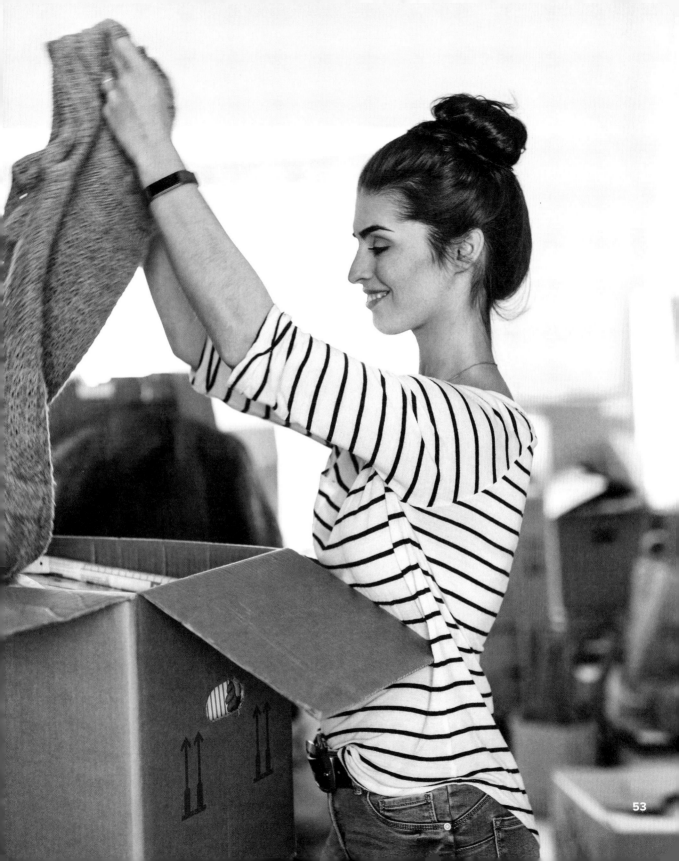

Most of us are familiar with Japanese author and organizing guru Marie Kondo and her take-no-prisoners approach of letting go of anything that doesn't "spark joy," but all that accumulated stuff affects us at a much more fundamental level. According to a 2011 Princeton University study, the chaos of a cluttered environment competes for our attention and limits our ability to focus and process information. In other words, clutter inhibits our conscious thinking and mindfulness.

"Mindfulness is all about finding balance without judgment," says Eva Selhub, MD, author of *The Stress Management Handbook*. "Decreasing clutter helps us feel more balanced, less distracted and more aware of our surroundings."

According to Chantale Bordonaro, founder and CEO of San Francisco-based organizing service Simplicity Source, decluttering isn't a one-size-fits-all proposition. What's "right" depends on what's most productive or efficient, given how you live or work. "If [your stuff] brings you down—affecting your space, your energy or your emotions—you need to address the problem," she says. "And anything that reduces anxiety and decreases stress creates good energy."

This idea is reinforced by a 2012 UCLA study that found that families who lived with a lot of clutter generally experienced high levels of cortisol, a stress hormone associated with chronic illness.

As Bordonaro points out, not only does decluttering lead to clearer thinking and less tension in our relationships, but not always having to look for what you need results in "found time," and positive energy that you can use to do new, different things. Ultimately, she says, decluttering makes you feel empowered. "You feel good because you gave yourself permission to take care of yourself and your space."

Finally, it's that awareness, realizing how good we feel that makes us want to keep doing it—or helps us realize we need to do it again. "Everyone is in search of 'happy' through outside means, such as buying things," says Selhub. "But really, it's all about finding happiness within ourselves and living in a balanced environment."

CREATING SPACE

How one woman found room for her life when she got rid of her excess stuff.

Patricia Desiderio, a school district administrator on the North Fork of Long Island, wasn't on a mission to thoroughly declutter her home when she and her husband recently embarked on a major renovation project. But what started as your average sorting-and-packing job soon took on other proportions once she realized how much space—mental and physical—the process created. "I started going through all my clothes very consciously," she says.

Because that felt so good, she began applying that same consciousness to every room in the house. "I made an effort to connect with what I wanted to keep, what I wanted to toss and what I decided to give away," she shares. "As I got going, I realized I was ridding myself of things that were weighing me down, even going through some things that have been in boxes since we moved in 17 years ago."

The end results of her whole-house decluttering efforts were even greater than she had anticipated. "I created all this new space—both literally and spiritually. Now I have room to think, write, meditate or to have a quiet cup of tea—I even think I'm sleeping better." Beyond that, she also has a new relationship with her clothes: "I got rid of so many things, it's really freeing." And what's left, "I'm seeing it with a fresh eye," she adds. Despite getting rid of so much, she feels like she has more things to wear. In the end, she says the whole process simply made her feel good. "For me, inner peace is a manifestation of my external space."

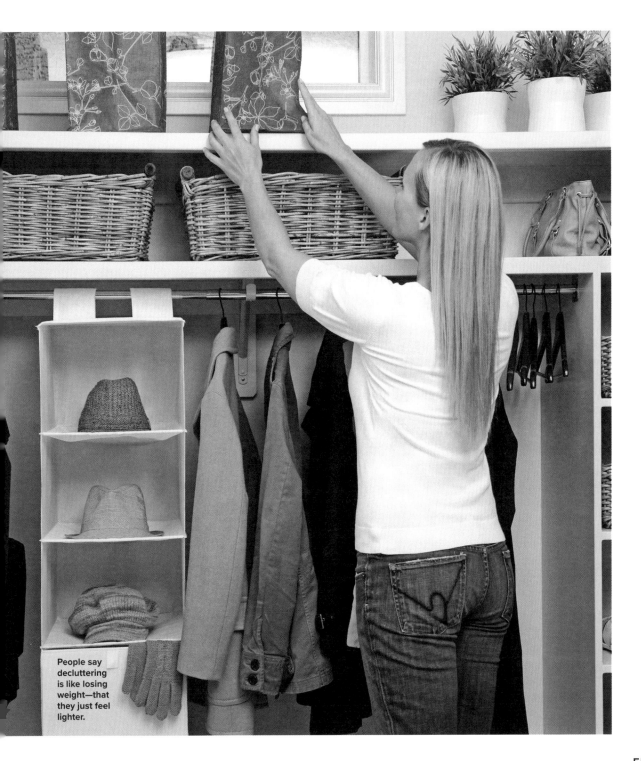

People say
decluttering
is like losing
weight—that
they just feel
lighter.

55

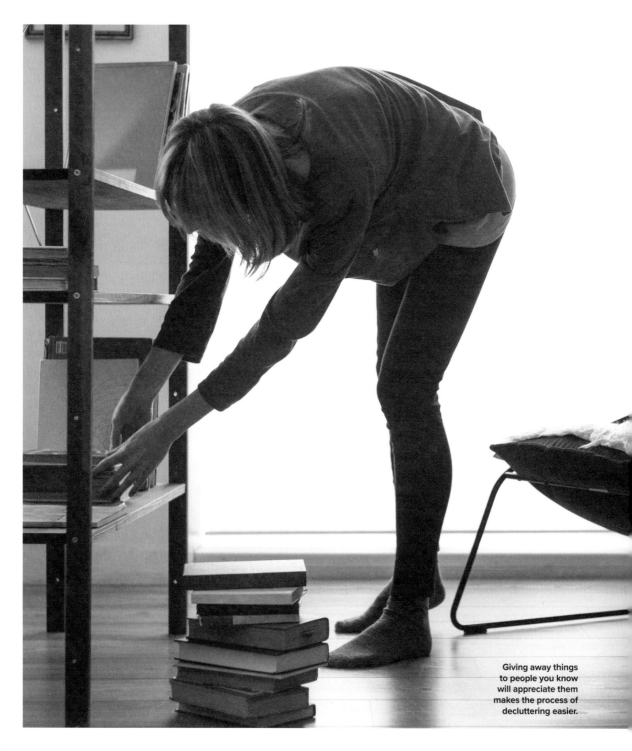

Giving away things to people you know will appreciate them makes the process of decluttering easier.

TIPS TO HELP YOU PARE DOWN

Before starting any decluttering project, professional organizer Chantale Bordonaro recommends setting realistic goals. It can be an exhausting process—physically and mentally—so pace yourself, and get help, if necessary. Keep in mind that you have to declutter before you can really start organizing. And finally, know that once you pull everything out it often gets worse before it gets better. Don't be discouraged, but be sure to finish one area before moving on to the next. Ready? Here are some of her tried-and-true tips:

→ START SMALL Begin with the easiest, most obvious things, the "low-hanging fruit"—the mess atop your desk, clothes that don't fit, toys your children have outgrown, old CDs, things you no longer use, etc. This helps you get focused, and builds confidence to start digging deeper.

→ FOCUS ON "EXPERIENCES" OVER "THINGS" "As your life changes, your environment also needs to keep evolving," says Bordonaro. What do you really want to keep and *why*? What's really important to you? Bordonaro points to one client who had a collection of old concert tickets and programs; ultimately she helped them scan everything and create a digital scrapbook, creating a new experience they could share with friends and family.

→ TRY A "30-DAY NO-SHOPPING CHALLENGE" Limit or stop shopping for non-essential items for a month. The goal: to better understand how and why you shop, and set priorities that make more sense, such as limiting bulk-buying or sticking with a "one piece in/one piece out" plan. Bordonaro also recommends keeping a small box in your closet for things you no longer want, so that decluttering becomes an ongoing process, and not something you only address occasionally.

→ FOLLOW THE 30 PERCENT RULE If a bookcase is stuffed full, for example, aim to take 30 percent of the books out. Not only will it look less jammed, but it will also be more inviting. "If you fill every space, you leave no room for energy to move around," says Bordonaro.

→ FIND A NEW HOME FOR THINGS Not everything needs to be thrown out. Is there an organization that could use some of your gently used things? Maybe you have a friend who's always coveted that item? Or a cousin whose young children can use your kids' hand-me-downs? "When you have a place or person in mind to give something to, it's a lot easier to let go," says Bordonaro.

→ CREATE A SYSTEM YOU CAN STICK WITH Whatever you're organizing, find the system that works best for how you live, work or think. Bordonaro often suggests clients buy uniform clothes hangers and then hang everything in the same direction. "Not only does it look neater, but it inspires you to want to keep it that way." For something like spices, think about how you use them. Some people organize alphabetically, some by flavor (salty or spicy) and others by cuisine type (e.g., Mexican versus Italian).

→ WORK WITH PROS If you have a big or emotionally difficult job ahead, such as cleaning out a childhood home, and you think you need help, you'll benefit from working with someone who has professional training. Certifications to look for: NAPO (National Assoc. of Productivity & Organizing Professionals; *napo.net*) and NASMM (National Assoc. of Senior Move Managers; *nasmm.org*).

CREATIVE MINDFULNESS

Crafts such as knitting,
drawing and even cooking can be
key parts of your practice.

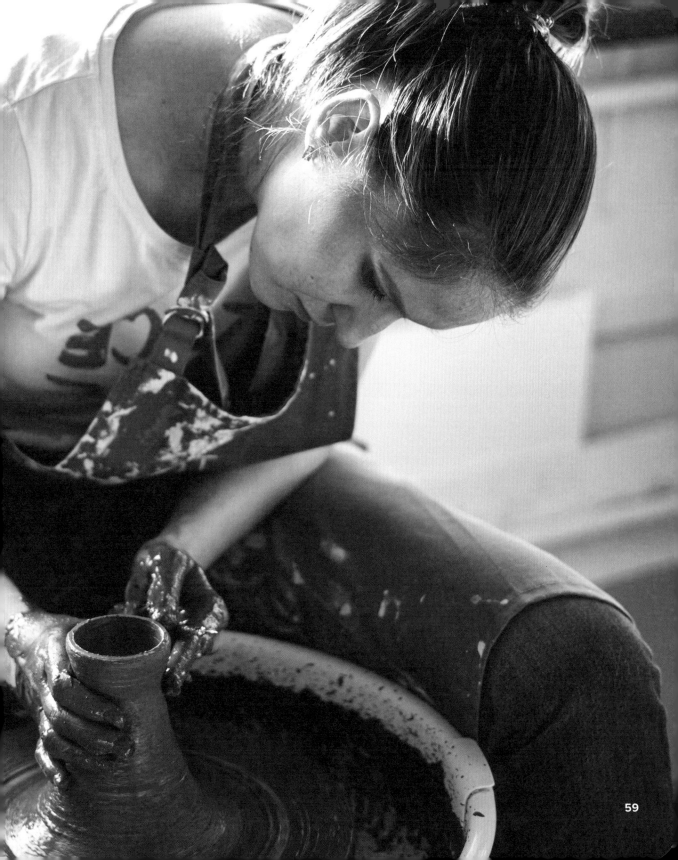

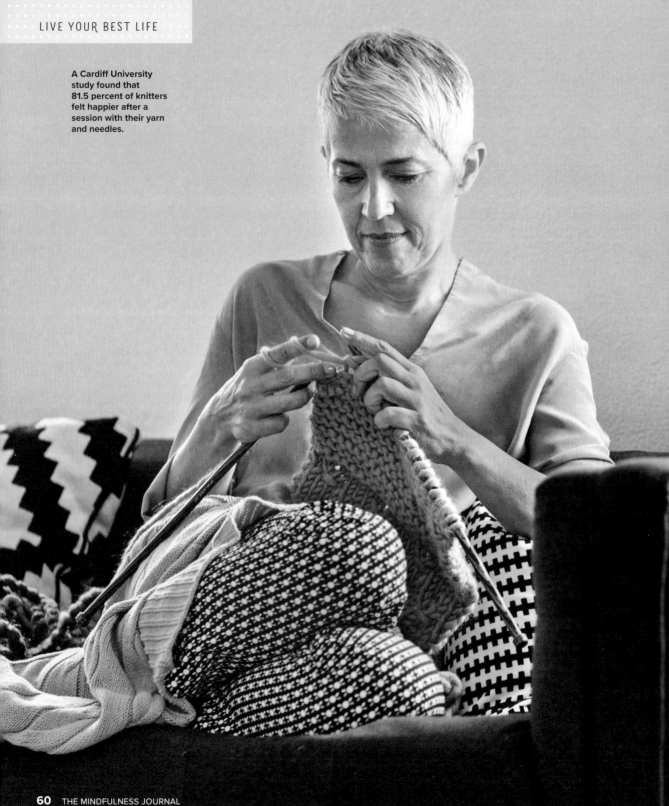

A Cardiff University study found that 81.5 percent of knitters felt happier after a session with their yarn and needles.

For some of us, starting a meditation practice is about as easy as learning to be a concert pianist. If you're one of these people, fear not! There is another path to mindfulness: creative activities. "Drawing, painting, knitting, sewing, coloring and other crafts where you use your mind and hands together can transport you into a state of mindfulness," says Christa Santangelo, PhD, a clinical psychologist and assistant clinical professor at the University of California, San Francisco. And there is an added bonus: These practices will result in an actual, often useful, product! The key is paying attention to the process. Take knitting: Focusing on the task combined with the repetitive hand motions can help lower your heart rate and blood pressure and bring about a relaxed state that is similar to meditation. It's also its own feedback loop: If you don't concentrate, the very tangible result is that you will make an obvious, visible mistake.

RESEARCH BACKS THIS UP

● Since the mid-1990s, hundreds of thousands of knitters and crocheters surveyed by the Craft Yarn Council have cited stress relief as a top reason for pursuing their crafts. And a study in the journal *Art Therapy* suggested that coloring "a reasonably complex geometric pattern may induce a meditative state." Drexel University researchers found that using collage materials, modeling clay and/or markers for 45 minutes lowered levels of the stress hormone cortisol in 75 percent of participants. And there's more: Other studies have shown that crafts can trigger the release of dopamine and serotonin, which improves feelings of well-being in the body.

Marygrace Berberian, MA, a clinical assistant professor of art therapy at NYU Steinhardt in New York City, agrees. "Creating art can be a good way to practice mindfulness," but, she adds, "it has to involve some intentionality." It's also important to pay attention to your senses. "What are you feeling, thinking, smelling, hearing? The key is to both notice the sensory elements and to focus," she adds. These factors can help bring about a state of what experts call flow. "When you're in flow, you are feeling immersed in the process, and you feel like you are transcending time and space. These are the experiences where we feel a deep sense of exhilaration," she says.

So how do you decide which craft is right for you? Berberian says that "some people will most benefit from stimulating their senses by diving into highly tactile activities like sculpting with clay or using really wet paint. Others—those who are soothed by maintaining a high level of control—find that they benefit more from the repetitive movements of crafts like knitting, sewing, crocheting or coloring."

"Experiment with different things to see what puts you in a state where you can have a sense of joy and ease and let go of judgment," Santangelo advises. "For some, it might be coloring; for others, cooking—or even just chopping garlic. Let the childlike part of you guide you to whatever feels right."

THE ZEN OF KNITTING

This popular hobby isn't just about expanding your wardrobe.

Knitting takes time, patience, a few supplies and some know-how. But along with keeping yourself and your loved ones cozy with homemade scarves, sweaters, hats and more, it can help you achieve a sense of mindfulness!

There is a veritable tapestry of instructional videos and articles available online to help you learn the basic stitches and provide you with patterns. For free instruction, try sheepandstitch.com; mybluprint.com offers a wide variety of crafting classes for a monthly fee of $7.99. Your local yarn store can be a great source of information—and, often, classes.

As you knit and purl, don't forget to focus on the sensations of your handiwork and on your breath. You will notice the thoughts that go through your mind, but gently return to the task at hand. Over time, you'll end up with both a useful hand-knit treasure and a mindfulness practice.

CONSCIOUS COOKING

Who knew making dinner could be mindful?

When psychologist Christa Santangelo, PhD, mentioned that cooking can be a form of mindfulness, I asked myself, could it be true? Could I meditate without a cushion and a gong? I decided to give it a whirl one night when I was home alone with no distractions.

I decided to make a dish that I ate often growing up: turkey tacos. I figured the fond childhood memories would somehow enhance the experience. But I also knew that the exercise wasn't about being in my head, but in the moment. "Allow yourself to be 100 percent present with the different physical senses, rather than being lost in thought," Andy Puddicombe, co-founder of the meditation app Headspace, wrote about mindful cooking in *Psychology Today*.

→ **THAT SOUNDED DOABLE** I fought the desire to turn on a podcast, my usual cooking soundtrack. I grabbed my favorite cast-iron skillet, noticing its weight. I put it on the burner, appreciating the clank of metal on metal. I turned on the gas, hearing the click of the lighter, then smelling a whiff of gas before blue flames started dancing below the iron. "Wow," I thought. "There is so much to notice!" Then

I detected some sort of brown substance in the middle of the pan. I grabbed a paper towel to rub it off and suddenly my mind was racing: "What is that stuff? Is it harmful? Have I ruined my skillet?"

I was only a minute in and already distraction, stress and judgment had reared their non-mindful heads. I remembered what Puddicombe had advised, took a deep breath and went back to the task at hand.

As I opened the package of ground turkey, I noted how the plastic slid off smoothly. As the meat hit the skillet, I heard it sizzle. I used a spatula to break it up and noticed how it began to change color, from pink to brownish-gray. Smoke began to rise toward me, and it smelled delicious.

→ **I GLANCED AT THE CLOCK** "I wonder how long this will take?" I thought. I began ruminating about how much I had to do before bedtime and, once again, I was out of the moment and in my head. "This is so frustrating!" I said out loud, causing my chihuahua to preemptively bark at whatever fear was threatening me. I laughed and then again heard Puddicombe's voice in my

head: "Each time the mind wanders, just bring the attention back to the sounds and smells."

→ **ALL RIGHT THEN** The meat was still sizzling and smelling delicious, but was now mostly brown. I added some seasoning and smiled as the rich spicy aroma swirled through the air. I breathed it all in and felt myself relax. Was this the elusive flow state? Was I in it? "I think I am in flow!" I thought, as I reminded myself to refocus.

I turned the flame down and began to grate the cheese, noticing how the slivers fell through each hole like graceful Olympic divers. Then I heated up a lovely, round tortilla, flipping it over with my fingers, noticing how hot it was, watching it begin to curl up a bit and become more pliable. I spooned some turkey into the middle, then added the cheese, which softened and began to melt. I inhaled the delicious scent and realized I wasn't thinking about how long this was taking, I was just enjoying the process. I topped my taco with salsa and lettuce and sat down at the table. I couldn't wait to eat my taco—hopefully in a mindful way.

—*Katherine Wessling*

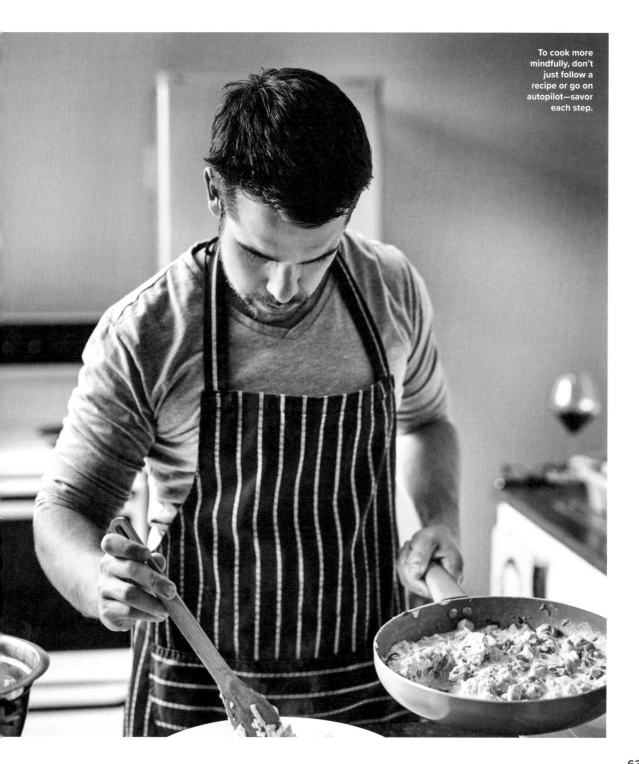

To cook more mindfully, don't just follow a recipe or go on autopilot—savor each step.

63

HELPING OTHERS, HELPING YOURSELF

Volunteering can be even more meaningful than doing downward-facing dog or a loving-kindness meditation.

When you hear the word mindfulness, practices like yoga, journaling and meditation are probably the first things that come to mind. But volunteering at a nearby food pantry or reading to children at your local library is another, especially meaningful way to cultivate it. "Any type of volunteering has a host of mindfulness benefits, including connecting you with others, alleviating isolation, providing purpose, lowering stress and enhancing your sense of gratitude in the process," says Gail Saltz, MD, a clinical associate professor of psychiatry at Weill-Cornell Medical College in New York. Best of all, any volunteer activity, for any amount of time, offers benefits, she adds. Intrigued? Read on.

HOW VOLUNTEERING BOOSTS MINDFULNESS

● Celebrity trainer Jillian Michaels knows firsthand the mindfulness benefits of volunteering. For the past two decades, she has been working with groups as diverse as Stand Up to Cancer and the United Nations. "Volunteering helps to bring meaning into my life, a greater sense of purpose, and helps me feel just a little less helpless," she says.

Research has long shown that volunteering boosts both your overall physical and emotional health: One 2017 analysis of over 40,000 people published in the medical journal *PLOS ONE*, for example, found that folks who regularly volunteer have fewer health problems than those who don't. "Volunteering is

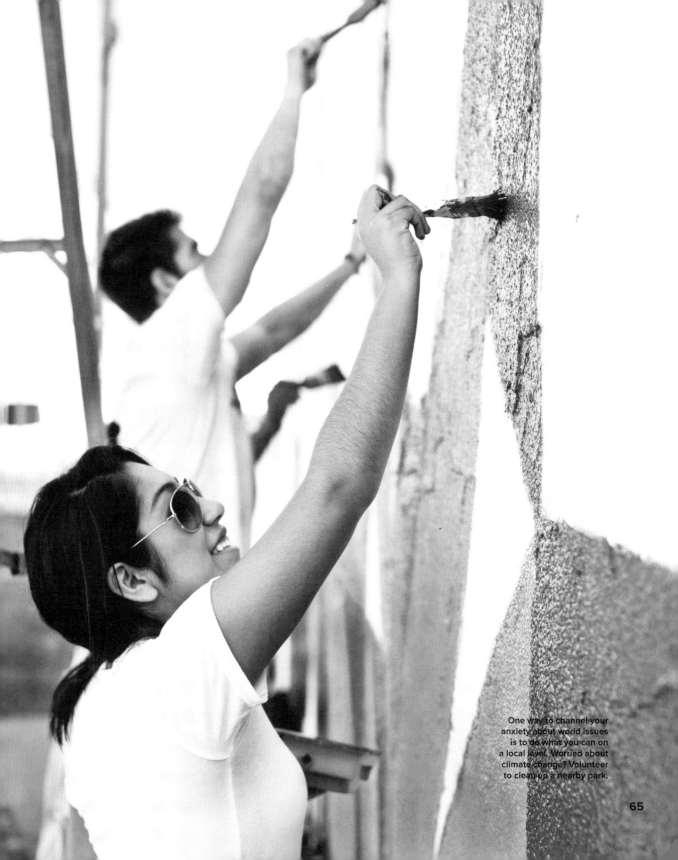

One way to channel your anxiety about world issues is to do what you can on a local level. Worried about climate change? Volunteer to clean up a nearby park.

a way to spark social connection, thus warding off loneliness and depression," explains Saltz.

Volunteering also provides a sense of happiness that boosts mood just as much as other activities such as talk therapy or exercise. The more adults volunteer, the happier they are, according to a London School of Economics study published in 2018 in the *British Journal of Industrial Relations*. Whether you are counseling single mothers at a shelter or picking up trash at a park, volunteering offers you a purpose that goes beyond the day-to-day grind of your work and personal life. "Finding something you're passionate about creates what I call a state of flow—you're doing something that makes you feel good, which boosts your mood," says Saltz. Here are some other ways helping the less fortunate boosts mindfulness:

IT CONNECTS YOU TO OTHERS When you volunteer, it forces you to focus on other people, which often provides a sense of purpose. "It allows us to remain fully present in the moment," explains Lynn Berger, LMHC, a licensed mental health counselor in New York City. "We start to think about how we're helping others, which makes us realize we have the power to make a positive impact on their lives."

It also allows you to become more engaged with communities that you might otherwise not interact with. This experience can promote mindfulness by making you realize that all people—regardless of race, ethnicity, socioeconomic class or nationality—are more alike than different. When Michaels recently visited the Democratic Republic of the Congo with the United Nations Refugee Agency, it was a life changer. "There's no Wi-Fi, no TV, nothing," she says. "Just yourself and the people with you—you had no choice but to be present and engaged."

IT CALMS YOUR MIND "We have so many thoughts racing through our minds at all times—I probably spend about half of my waking day 'time traveling,' thinking about what I could have done better in the past or what I need to do differently for tomorrow," says Michaels. Volunteering, on the other hand, demands that you be present enough to concentrate

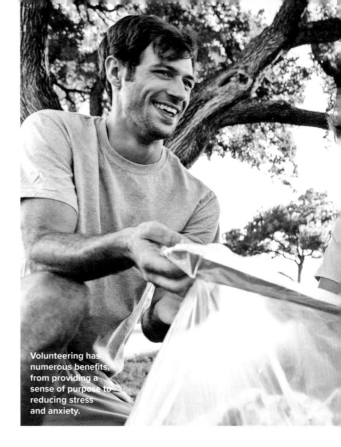

Volunteering has numerous benefits, from providing a sense of purpose to reducing stress and anxiety.

on the task at hand. "That reason in itself helps to combat the stress and anxiety of regretting yesterday or worrying about tomorrow," she adds.

In today's world, where it's normal to feel overwhelmed and helpless when it comes to global problems like climate change, volunteering can help relieve anxiety. Rather than ruminating, you can channel your worry into something positive, like becoming involved with a nonprofit environmental group. "This in turn lowers stress hormones such as adrenaline and cortisol that contribute to anxiety," explains Saltz. Case in point: A 2013 Carnegie Mellon University study found that adults who volunteered on a regular basis were less likely to develop high blood pressure—which is often triggered by stress— than non-volunteers.

IT GIVES YOU PERSPECTIVE Volunteering helps you gain empathy and insight, two valuable mindfulness tools. "When we connect to something

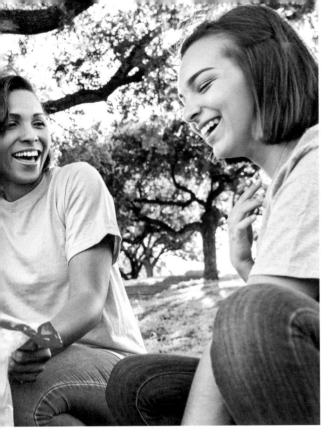

bigger than ourselves, it helps us to see our own issues from a different perspective," says Salina Shelton, LPC, a licensed professional counselor and art therapist in San Antonio. "Suddenly our problems might not seem as bad."

The ability to really stand in another person's shoes and feel grateful for what you have in life also gives you a sense of agency and power. "You've giving to others, which in turn makes you feel good and allows you to be mindful and present as positive things are going on," adds Saltz.

IT INCREASES SELF-CONFIDENCE When you do good for others, you gain a sense of accomplishment that makes you feel good about yourself. And the better you feel about yourself, the more likely you are to believe your life has meaning. Altruistic people—those who have genuine concern about the well-being of others—tend to be happiest overall, according to a 2010 Harvard Business School survey.

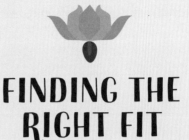

FINDING THE RIGHT FIT

Volunteering will be more fulfilling if you find the right mission.

Volunteering is like exercise: You need to enjoy it to stay motivated and keep doing it. Here are some keys for getting started—and sticking with it.

→ **START SMALL** Your first volunteer job shouldn't be becoming a foster parent or building wells in Africa—it's likely you'll quickly get overwhelmed and drop out. "There are so many things you can do—like run a charity 5K—that are a one-off," says psychiatrist Gail Saltz. Once you've dipped your toe into the water, commit to a time frame that is realistic and reasonable for you. "If two hours a week is too much, try every other week, or once a month," says art therapist Salina Shelton. "If you overcommit, you run the risk of burnout and may not enjoy it as much."

→ **BE STRATEGIC** Pick something that you actually have an interest in. Maybe you love animals, so walking pups at a shelter is a natural choice. Or your father benefited from the care he received at the local hospital, and you want to pay it back. Torn between several? Choose a different cause each month and set a goal to give back at least once a month until you determine what you're most passionate about, advises Nicole Black, a former teacher in Agoura Hills, California, who runs the blog Coffee and Carpool: Raising Kind Kids.

→ **MAKE IT A FAMILY AFFAIR** Whenever possible, bring your spouse and even your kids along—it's a way to connect as a family. "It imbues even more meaning into the activity, since you'll need to explain to your children why you're volunteering—who it helps, what it does," adds Saltz. It also exposes them to a wider range of people.

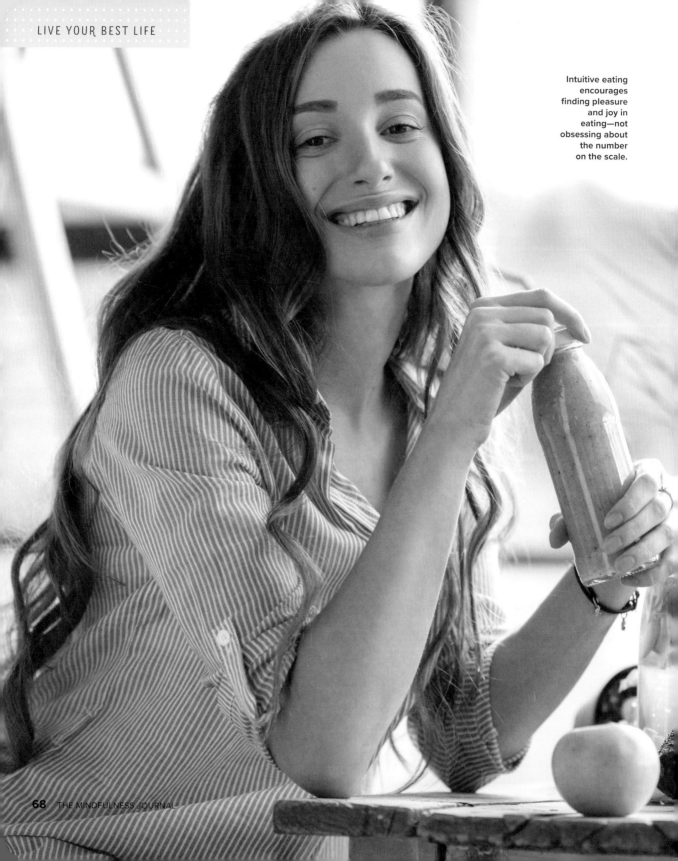

Intuitive eating encourages finding pleasure and joy in eating—not obsessing about the number on the scale.

GETTING
IN TUNE

If thinking about food—what to eat, when to dine and feeling guilty about less-than-healthy meals—is taking up too much of your mental bandwidth, intuitive eating may be for you.

These days, it seems that everywhere you look, from Instagram to your inbox —even on the nightly newscasts—there's something or someone touting the benefits of a new, better, healthier way to eat. Whether that means drinking gallons of celery juice, eating just a few hours a day or hopping on the #keto bandwagon, it's clear that our society believes the right diet is the path to wellness.

Given that we're all individuals with a unique amalgamation of genetics and environmental influences, how do you know which is the "right" diet for *you*? Considering the amount of money Americans spend on diet programs each year, it's safe to say that's the $1 million—er, $60 billion— question. But what if the solution to healthy eating wasn't actually a diet. What if the answer was actually in our minds?

Well, that's precisely what two pioneering dieticians, Evelyn Tribole and Elyse Resch, sought to impart back in 1995, in a groundbreaking book, *Intuitive Eating: A Revolutionary Program That Works*. Since then, intuitive eating has become "a scientifically studied, evidence-based paradigm that helps you connect with your body's inner wisdom to determine what to eat, how much to eat and when to eat," explains Kara Lydon, RD, LDN, a certified intuitive eating counselor and owner of Kara Lydon Nutrition. "It's different from a diet, in that you are not following a list of external rules (e.g., cut out X food or don't eat past X time), but rather honoring your body's own internal cues and focusing on more gentle guidelines as they pertain to nutrition and health."

Today, the culture-changing work of Tribole and Resch is celebrated by reformed dieters around the world—and its efficacy is supported by a growing body of scientific literature. "Studies have shown that intuitive eating is associated with higher levels of body appreciation, self-esteem and satisfaction with life, and lower levels of eating disorder behaviors, body-checking and body shame," says Lydon, who's also a yoga teacher. "Intuitive eating has also been associated with a lower BMI; however, weight loss is not the intended outcome of intuitive eating."

Cases in point: A 2018 study in the *American Journal of Health Promotion* found that the Health at Every Size (HAES) intervention—which includes mindful eating—helped women battling weight and body-image issues improve variables such as weight, eating behaviors and emotional well-being. Research in the journal *Eating Behaviors* in 2017 reported that intuitive eating was directly linked with decreased levels of disordered eating and better body image. A 2016 review in *Nutrition Research Reviews* discovered that it was also the most effective way of overcoming binge eating and emotional eating. (For a full listing of studies, visit intuitiveeating.org.)

A RULE-FREE ZONE

● Think of intuitive eating as a blueprint for how to establish a healthy and sustainable relationship with food, Lydon says. "Rather than a set of rules, it offers guidelines or tools that you can use when you need them. Since there are no rules, there's no failing, either—only opportunities for learning more about your body."

Intuitive eating is founded on the principles Tribole and Resch outline in their book, including:

Honoring your body's internal hunger/fullness cues

Making peace with all foods (meaning there are no "good" or "bad" foods)

Honoring your cravings

Rejecting diet culture, including fad diets and food trends

Respecting your body

Engaging in joyful movement (i.e., doing exercise you enjoy, not slogging through the "it" class of the moment)

Although mindful eating doesn't restrict food groups or promote weight loss, that doesn't mean that nutrition is off the menu. "Because intuitive eating is often depicted on Instagram with photos of burgers and pizza, people automatically assume that intuitive eating doesn't care about nutrition or health, but it's quite the opposite," Lydon says. When you tune in to how your body feels, you may start "craving" foods like fruits, vegetables, whole grains and legumes that leave you feeling satisfied and invigorated, not bloated and tired (like after eating candy and chips).

Another way to look at it, according to Lydon: "With intuitive eating, you're not only choosing what foods *sound* good to you in the moment, but also tapping into your body's wisdom of what is going to *feel* good in the moment. Some days that might be pizza, and other days that might be a salad."

WORTH ITS WEIGHT

● Even though it's true some people might naturally lose weight when paying close attention to their internal body cues and honoring their fullness level, dropping pounds isn't the end game here—far from it.

"Unlike diets that are intended for intentional weight loss, intuitive eating is centered around establishing a sustainable relationship with food and health that doesn't compromise your mental or emotional well-being," notes Lydon. "Although weight loss can happen as a result of intuitive eating, it can also result in weight maintenance or weight gain, depending on the individual."

If you're someone who has struggled with an eating disorder—which may have been provoked in part by trying to lose weight—intuitive eating can be particularly helpful. "Intuitive eating is often utilized in the treatment of eating disorders, to help people fully recover and heal," Lydon says. "However, it's important for those struggling with an eating

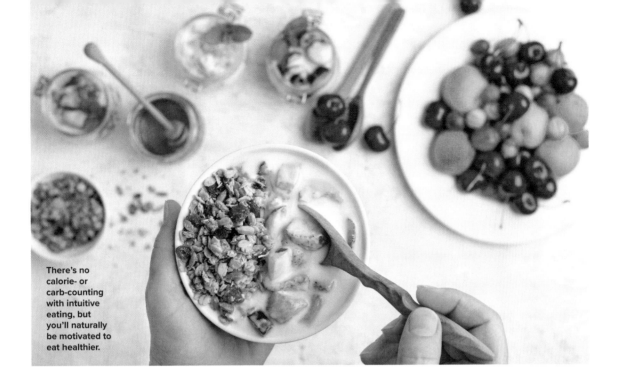

There's no calorie- or carb-counting with intuitive eating, but you'll naturally be motivated to eat healthier.

disorder to seek out professional help, because those who are undernourished will often have unreliable internal cues and will benefit from more structure."

BREAKING FREE

• Intuitive eating paves the way for food freedom, Lydon shares. "Many of my clients come to me complaining that they think about food all day long; that it is utterly exhausting, as they have no bandwidth left for anything else. When you make peace with food and heal your relationship with it through intuitive eating, it frees up so much mental space for your values and things that you actually want to be focusing on, like career, relationships and hobbies."

Another upside: "Intuitive eating helps to take the morality and black-and-white thinking out of food," Lydon says. "It creates so much more room for satisfaction and finding pleasure in food, and in turn reduces anxiety and distress around eating."

GETTING STARTED

• While eating intuitively may sound simple, if you've been dieting most of your life, it might be tricky

at first. "I highly recommend finding a certified intuitive eating dietitian (you can find one at intuitiveeating.org) or therapist to work with to help support you in your intuitive eating journey," Lydon advises.

In the meantime, to help get a flavor for what it means to be more mindful at mealtime and throughout your day, heed Lydon's advice: "Start by noticing the satisfaction factor of foods: What foods satisfy you on both a physical and mental level? When you are making a choice about what to eat, ask yourself, what temperature, texture, volume and flavor of food sounds the most satisfying to me right now?"

One thing's for sure: You absolutely have permission to eat that pizza—but be sure to take a moment to smell the freshly baked crust, to savor the salty cheese mixed with the sweet tomato sauce. And before you dig in, you also want to reflect on how you much you would enjoy—and how good you would feel—if you decided to eat a salad, a bowl of tomato soup or a crispy apple instead. However, if pizza is what you're craving, enjoy it guilt-free. That's the whole point of intuitive eating.

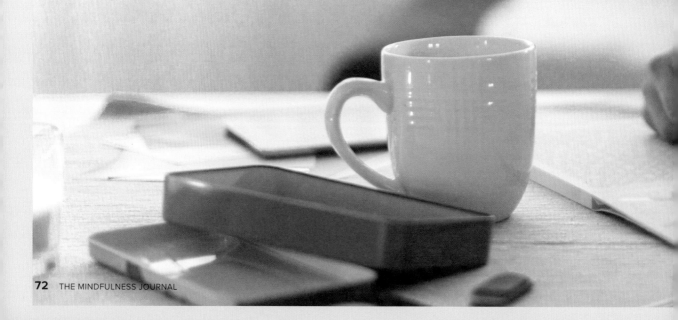

PART 2

express YOURSELF

Mindfulness is not just meditation
and yoga—keeping a journal can
help you sort out your goals and emotions,
and live a more content life.

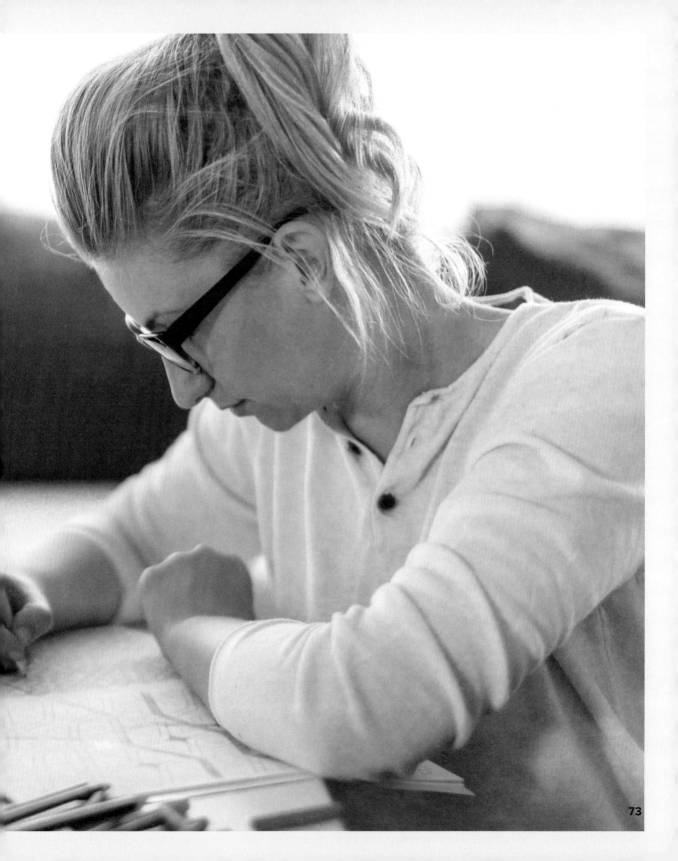

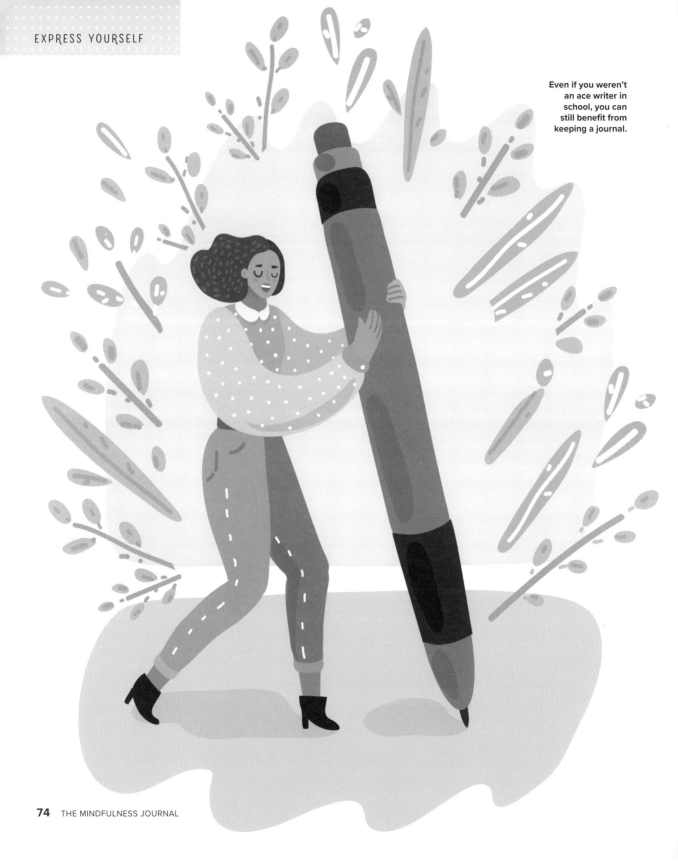

Even if you weren't an ace writer in school, you can still benefit from keeping a journal.

THE JOYS OF
JOURNALING

Putting pen to paper can help you gain
perspective on your life, reduce stress,
heal trauma and boost resilience.

You probably write a lot, every day: Texts. Emails. Reports. Facebook and Twitter posts. And it's likely that most, if not all, of those words are outward-facing: "Meeting at 4 in the conference room." "Preliminary notes on September project." Meanwhile, our own inner selves are often far in the background. Our words are all about the future, planning, organizing. We are constantly checking in with others, but rarely checking in with ourselves.

Now imagine taking just a few minutes of that writing time each day to focus on only one thing: You. Not your schedule, or posting on Instagram about your latest vacation, but simply what's going on in your head. It's called journaling, and it's been helping people understand themselves and their lives for centuries, says Maud Purcell, MSW, LCSW, CEAP, a psychotherapist and founder of The Life Solution Center in Darien, Connecticut. "Journaling is an ancient tradition that dates back to at least 10th-century Japan," says Purcell. "Successful people throughout history have kept journals, from presidents to artists."

Journaling is garnering renewed attention now, as people look for ways to become more mindful and aware in their daily lives. The ties between writing in a journal and developing mindfulness are powerful. The very act of writing places you fully in the present, forcing you to put aside all that multitasking and focus inward—in a way that's similar to meditation and its focus on being present in the moment. In fact, some people consider journaling almost another form of meditation. And as in meditation, putting pen to paper by definition inserts some distance between the here-and-now and your over-busy brain that's reeling with thoughts and emotions. Rather than reacting to your inner swirl of feelings, you are simply recording and examining what's going on in there. Author and essayist Joan Didion once told an interviewer she had been keeping notebooks since the age of 5. She summed up the resulting clarity this way: "I don't know what I think until I write it down."

That clarity, and the process of being in the moment, is only the tip of the iceberg when it comes

FILL YOUR PAPER WITH THE BREATHINGS OF YOUR HEART."

WILLIAM WORDSWORTH

to the benefits of journaling, however. Research is showing concrete effects, both physical and psychological, of regularly writing in a journal. Here are some of the most encouraging findings.

IT HELPS HEAL TRAUMA

• A growing body of scientific literature has shown that writing about traumatic or stressful events can improve both physical and emotional health. For instance, a meta-analysis published in the journal *Advances in Psychiatric Treatment* looked at 20 years of studies. It found that when people were tasked with writing about upsetting events for 15 to 20 minutes on three to five occasions, they later had significantly better physical and psychological outcomes than people who wrote about neutral topics. While there was sometimes a short-term negative effect—an uptick in distress and a drop in mood—a longer-term follow-up showed ongoing benefits, including a greater sense of well-being, happier mood, fewer stress-related doctor visits, lower blood pressure and even improvements in working memory.

"The actual writing is in many ways beside the point," says Erica Leibrandt, LPC, RYT, a psychotherapist based in Glenview, Illinois. "What's important is that you begin to take ownership of your story." She knows about journaling from personal experience: While recovering from an abusive relationship, she wrote 500 pages over two years. "I was unintentionally doing something called

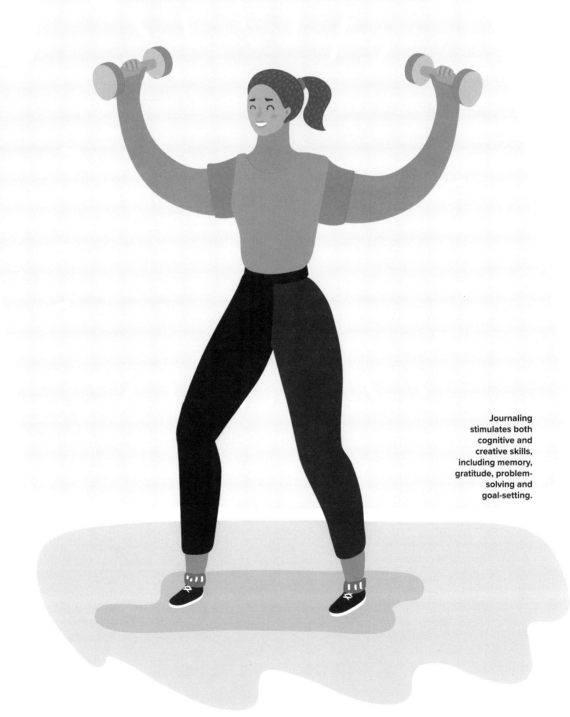

Journaling stimulates both cognitive and creative skills, including memory, gratitude, problem-solving and goal-setting.

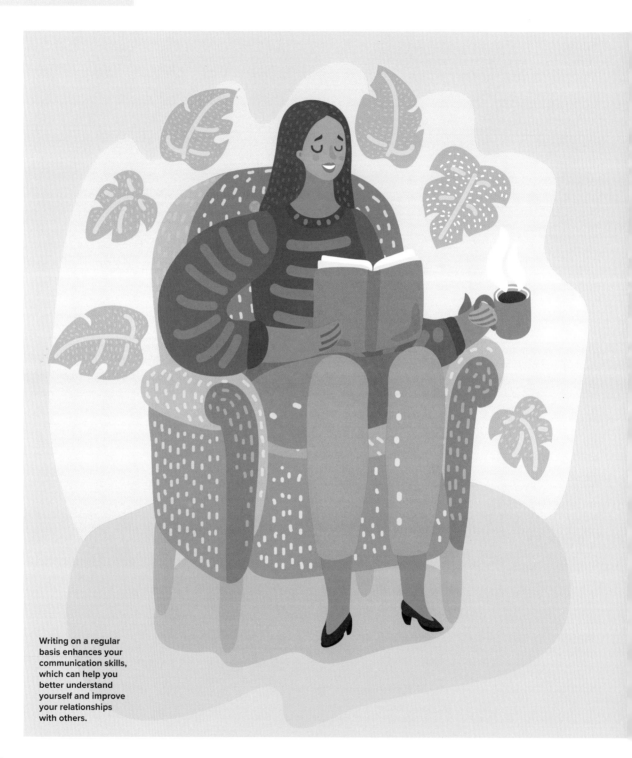

Writing on a regular basis enhances your communication skills, which can help you better understand yourself and improve your relationships with others.

GETTING STARTED

Want to reap the benefits of journaling? Here's how:

"The most important rule of all is that there are no rules," says psychotherapist Maud Purcell. That said, certain guidelines can help you get started and stay on track. Here's how:

→ **FIND THE RIGHT TOOLS** While it's certainly possible to write journal entries on a computer or mobile device, research suggests that old-fashioned pen and paper may be more effective. That's because they trigger the brain's reticular activating system, a network of neural pathways that connects the spinal cord with the cerebrum and cerebellum areas of the brain, which filter out distractions and enhance your focus. "Look for a notebook and writing implement that speak to you," says Purcell. "Then set up a journaling 'nook' with things that engage your senses, like fresh flowers or scented candles."

→ **START SMALL, BUT STEADY** Begin with a four-day writing exercise, suggests Shilagh Mirgain, PhD, a psychologist at the University of Wisconsin School of Medicine and Public Health. (Her guidelines are based on the work of James Pennebaker, PhD, who has conducted numerous studies

on the effects of journaling.) "Limit your writing to 15 to 20 minutes per session, but do try to write for four consecutive days, and keep at it until your time is up. If you run out of things to say before that, you can even repeat what you've already written." The act itself is part of the process.

→ **WRITE ABOUT ANYTHING YOU WANT** "You could write about something that's bothering you, or something very personal and important to you," says Mirgain. "Just trust where your writing takes you." One idea that can help free you, she adds, is to "remember that you're only writing for yourself, so don't hold back, and be as open and honest with yourself as possible. You could even decide to eventually destroy what you've written." If you feel stuck, try picking a theme for the day, week or month, suggests Purcell—"for example, peace of mind, confusion, change or anger."

→ **DON'T SWEAT THE DETAILS** "Let the pen and paper, rather than your rational brain, do the writing," says Purcell. "Don't feel constrained by proper grammar or punctuation, and write quickly.

This frees your brain from 'shoulds' and other blocks."

→ **KNOW WHEN TO STOP** If you find yourself struggling to write about something because it feels too upsetting, then don't, says Mirgain. "It may be a sign that you're not quite ready to explore that subject. Instead, start by focusing on situations or events that you feel you can handle." Eventually, you may surprise yourself with what emerges. "You can write your way to a new chapter," Mirgain adds. "Journaling reminds you that you alone are the author of your life story, and you have the power to say 'my journey has just begun.'"

→ **JOURNAL FIRST THING IN THE MORNING—OR RIGHT BEFORE BED** The time of day doesn't matter, Mirgain says. "If you don't want to take your worries to bed, write about your concerns for a few minutes at bedtime. This can improve your sleep. For other people, it may be preferable to journal in the morning. Starting the day with a few minutes of journaling will clear the clutter out of your head, so you can greet the day with a fresh perspective."

narrative therapy, and the benefits were remarkable," Leibrandt says now. A decade after that experience, and having become a psychotherapist, she went on to form a Write Club for clients who wanted to try journaling. "After the first session, I drove home ecstatic. It felt like months of therapeutic work had been accomplished in the space of a few hours. It was therapy on steroids!"

IT STRENGTHENS
THE IMMUNE SYSTEM

• Chronic stress or worry can increase the body's levels of hormones such as cortisol, the "fight-or-flight" chemical. While that's good when you're being threatened by immediate danger, when cortisol stays elevated over time it can suppress your immune system and cause damage throughout your body. A study in the *British Journal of Health Psychology* found that writing about an emotional topic lowered participants' cortisol levels. Other studies have shown that people had a more robust immune response to vaccinations after several sessions of writing about emotional events, and a 2013 study found that 76 percent of adults who spent 20 minutes writing about their thoughts and feelings for three days before getting a biopsy were fully healed 11 days later. Only 42 percent of the control group, who hadn't journaled, had gone back to normal in that time.

IT IMPROVES
FUTURE RESILIENCE

• Not only does journaling help you process events via the act of writing, it also offers emotional support for the future. "Journaling about past events reminds us powerfully that we've gotten through difficulties before," explains Purcell, "and with that comes hope and optimism. When a current dilemma seems insurmountable, you can look back on previous ones that you were able to resolve." Leibrandt's Write Club clients find that the emotional "digging" they do through journaling gives them fodder for more self-understanding, she says. "It excavates all kinds of psychological fossils that can continue to be examined long after the group has ended." The

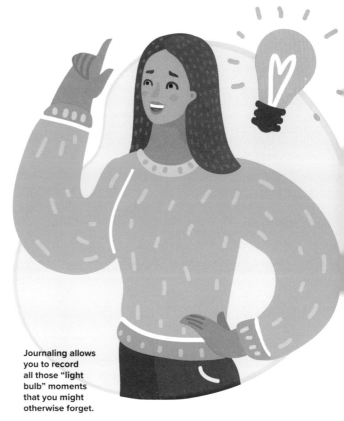

Journaling allows you to record all those "light bulb" moments that you might otherwise forget.

result: more effective therapy in the moment, and better emotional functioning in the future.

Journaling may achieve that partly through controlling the intensity of your emotions, enabling you to approach problems more rationally. Researchers at UCLA did brain scans on volunteers who journaled 20 minutes a day for four days, and found increased activity in the part of the prefrontal cortex, which works to regulate strong emotional feelings.

IT BOOSTS CREATIVITY

• "The act of writing accesses the left hemisphere of the brain, which is analytical and rational," says Purcell. "While your left brain is occupied, your right brain is free to create, intuit and feel. In this way, writing can remove mental blocks and allow you to use all of your brain power to better understand yourself, others and the world around you."

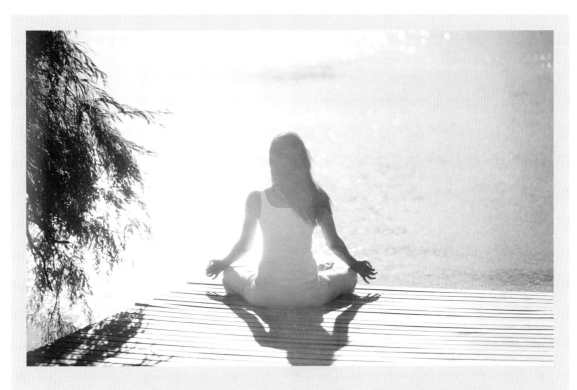

HOW MEDITATION ENHANCED MY JOURNALING

Combining the two practices can boost the mindfulness payoff.

Seven years ago, my daughter was diagnosed with a life-threatening illness. During those dark days, my thoughts were swirling, at times incoherent with internal chatter. My meditation teacher once told me that confusion is the beginning of understanding, and that awareness could help bring some clarity. Beginning when I was a teen, journaling has always brought me solace, allowing me the space to put emotions and expectations into perspective. So I decided to make meditation part of my journaling process.

Ever since then, just before bed, I meditate for 20 minutes and then journal for 20 minutes. My meditation always begins with a brief body-space awareness practice. Then I ask myself a question and just sit with it. I liken it to scooping a glass of water out of the river. If you set the glass down, the sediment will settle and the water will clear. This allows my brain to get to a place far deeper than mere thought usually allows, improving my focus and allowing me to think about profound things in a more imaginative way. I even take a paper and pen to my meditation cushion to jot down ideas that may pop up.

Journaling after this kind of brief meditation allows me to organize my thoughts before I start writing. When I first began, it helped me to care for my daughter in a more sympathetic and grounded way. Even after she got better, I found that combining the two practices was so powerful that I've continued ever since, though now my journaling tends toward compassion and gratitude, not only for my daughter's recovery, but for all beings.

—Sandra Fernandez

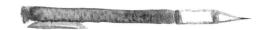

THE ABCs OF BULLET JOURNALING

This technique, embraced by everyone from artists to execs, is a great alternative to traditional diaries, while delivering many of the same benefits.

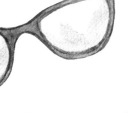

In our time-crunched, tech-fatigued world, many espouse the benefits of journaling to unplug and focus the mind. As a journalist by trade, I never considered that adding additional writing to my hectic daily schedule could enhance my productivity and mindfulness, helping me get more out of my career, motherhood and even my daily yoga/meditation practice.

But then I heard about bullet journaling. The brainchild of Ryder Carroll—author of *The Bullet Journal Method: Track the Past, Order the Present, Design the Future*—it's a thought-provoking method beloved by CEOs and stay-at-home moms alike. It helps people declutter their minds and live with intention via the daily practice of putting pen to paper.

But bullet journaling (aka BuJo), is a different animal than open-ended journaling, as it combines bulleted to-do lists, notes, reflections and goals in a simple organizational system that is customized by each individual. "It's a foundation that is designed to be modified by the user to meet their specific needs," explains Carroll, a New York–based designer.

BuJo not only helps people organize *what* they're doing, but it helps them clarify *why* they're doing it in the first place. With a busy schedule in the months ahead, I was clearly in need of an overhaul and dove right into BuJo. The return to handwriting felt warm and familiar. (In fact, scientific studies show that old-school, analog writing enhances memory; it forces us to slow down, allowing us to

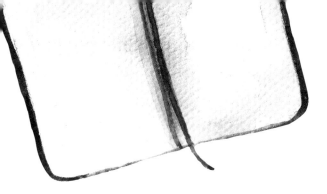
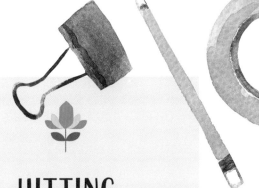

reflect on our life experiences and aspirations with a deeper sense of awareness.)

RETHINKING OBLIGATIONS

• Bullet journaling uses graphic signifiers—such as bullets, dots, right and left arrows—to categorize and prioritize tasks and events, as well as long-term goals, into one journal.

One of the bullet journal techniques I found most helpful is what Carroll calls Migration, in which you transfer commitments from page to page. It's one of the multiple filters you can use to "curate" your list on an ongoing basis, making sure that essential things don't fall through the cracks; at the same time, it forces you to continually re-evaluate what's important to you and allows you to let go of things that no longer matter. Carroll recommends committing to bullet journaling for at least two to three months to fully experience the Migration process.

Over time, I started discovering that the writing process made me prioritize tasks, shedding the ones that simply didn't matter anymore. I found myself more organized, which liberated my mind from anxiety and allowed me to be more mindful in choosing what I wanted to spend my time doing. "When people see how much they *don't* have to do, and that they get to decide what matters, that can be a very powerful experience." Carroll says.

A WORLDWIDE PHENOMENON

• On Instagram, people from all over the world have posted images of their bullet journals, some of which are stunningly creative. However, Carroll emphasizes that you shouldn't become intimidated by them. "It can be that, but it does not need to be," he says. Whether it's minimal or artistic, your bullet journal practice can be whatever you need it to be. —*Tess Ghilaga*

HITTING THE TARGET

Inventor Ryder Carroll provides some essential tips to creating a bullet journal that will help you get more organized, reduce stress and live a more mindful, meaningful life:

1

Before you begin, define what your challenge or aspiration is and what you want to get out of it.

2

To start your bullet journal, watch the step-by-step free tutorial on bulletjournal.com. Buy a high-quality notebook, and remember to index and number your pages (the tutorial and Carroll's book, *The Bullet Journal Method*, explain how). Or, you can purchase a numbered bullet journal online.

3

Use BuJo as a vehicle for self-learning. At first, keep it as simple as you need to, and be patient with yourself.

4

In your AM and PM Daily Log, review your lists on a daily basis to curate them.

5

At the end of each month, scan all the pages of the month to see how much you've accomplished with your tasks.

becoming more
MINDFUL

Why do you want to become more mindful?

_____

_____

_____

_____

_____

_____

_____

How do you think it will improve your life?

_____

_____

_____

_____

What steps are you going to take to help make it happen?

_____

_____

_____

_____

why you want to
JOURNAL

Write a list of your journaling goals.
Do you want to gain some perspective on your life?
Set goals? Understand your emotions?

_____

_____

_____

_____

_____

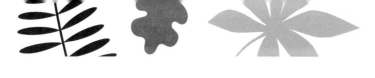

When do you plan on journaling
(how many times a week/what time of day)?

_____

_____

_____

_____

_____

_____

What are some obstacles you have faced in making
journaling a habit in the past?

_____

_____

_____

_____

_____

_____

How can you overcome them?

_____

_____

_____

contemplating NATURE

"THOSE WHO CONTEMPLATE THE BEAUTY OF THE EARTH FIND RESERVES OF STRENGTH THAT WILL ENDURE AS LONG AS LIFE LASTS."
RACHEL CARSON

What or where is your favorite view of nature?

_____

_____

_____

_____

_____

What feelings does that view evoke?

_____

_____

What's your favorite smell of the outdoors?

_____

What memories are associated with it?

_____

What are three ways you can spend more time outdoors?

_____

your BEST DAY ever

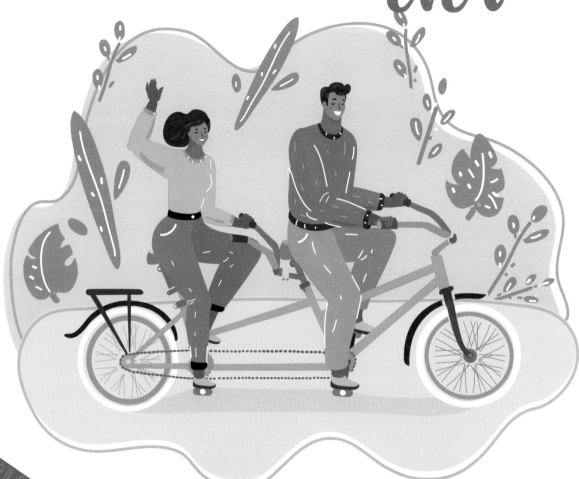

What would you do if you had
no obligations except to do your favorite things?

_____

_____

_____

_____

_____

_____

Who would you spend that day with?

_____

_____

_____

_____

_____

Where would you be?

_____

_____

_____

_____

rediscovering your
INNER CHILD

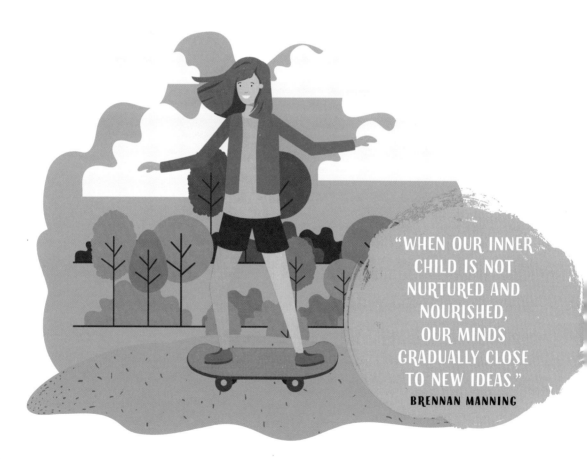

"WHEN OUR INNER CHILD IS NOT NURTURED AND NOURISHED, OUR MINDS GRADUALLY CLOSE TO NEW IDEAS."
BRENNAN MANNING

What five activities gave you the most pleasure as a kid?

_____

_____

_____

_____

_____

_____

What did you love about them?

_____

_____

_____

_____

_____

_____

What can you do to recapture some of that joy today?

_____

_____

_____

facing
YOUR
FEARS

What are your five greatest fears? Rate them each on a scale of one (very unlikely) to 10 (very likely) based on how likely they are to happen.

1 _____

_____

2 _____

_____

3 _____

_____

4 _____

_____

5 _____

_____

How has worrying had a negative impact on your life?

_____

_____

_____

_____

you're the
BEST

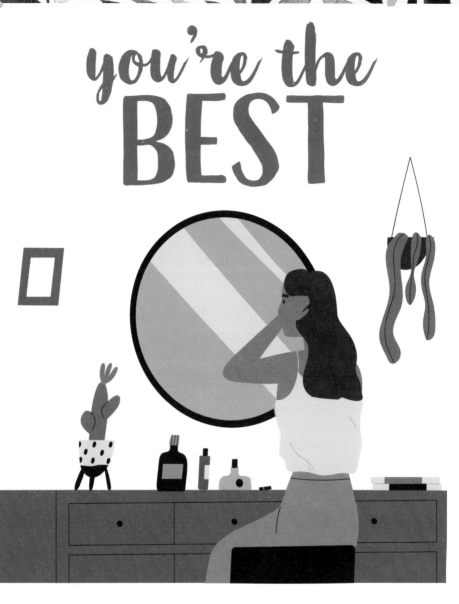

List your 10 favorite things about yourself. Why do you value each of them?

1 _____

_____

2

3

4

5

6

7

8

9

10

the joy of
SILENCE

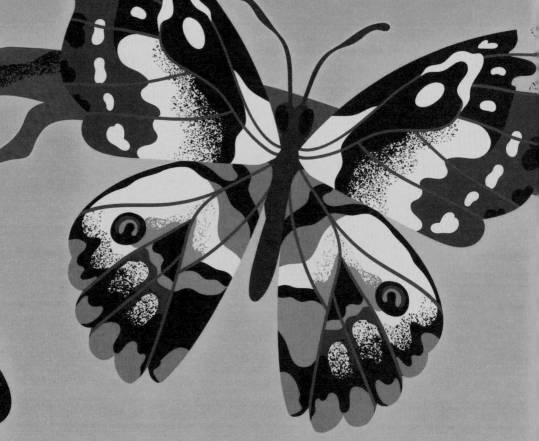

Turn off all devices and TVs for at least 10 minutes —just sit still and observe the world around you. What did you notice that you hadn't before?

_____

_____

_____

_____

_____

Do you feel like you missed anything? Would you like more of that calm in your life?

_____

_____

_____

_____

_____

_____

_____

_____

the perfect
MOMENT

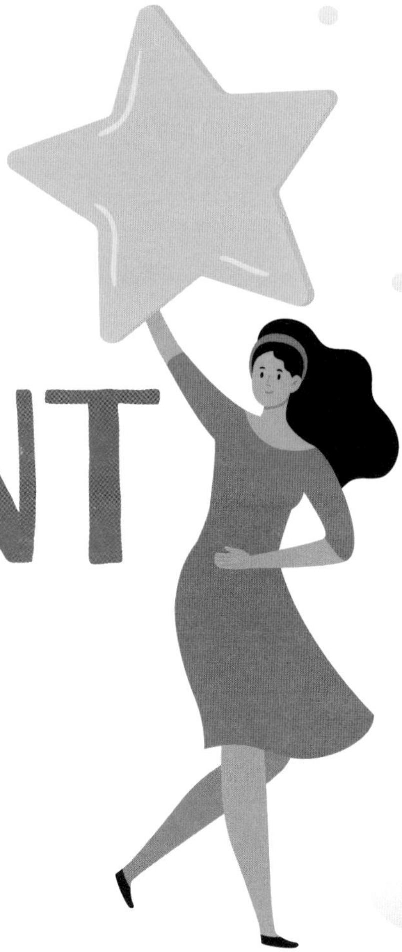

What is something you've always wanted to do?

_____

_____

_____

_____

_____

_____

Why have you been putting it off?

_____
_____
_____
_____
_____
_____

Is there a realistic way for you to get started right now? What would that look like?

_____
_____
_____
_____
_____
_____

How would it change the way you view your life?

_____
_____

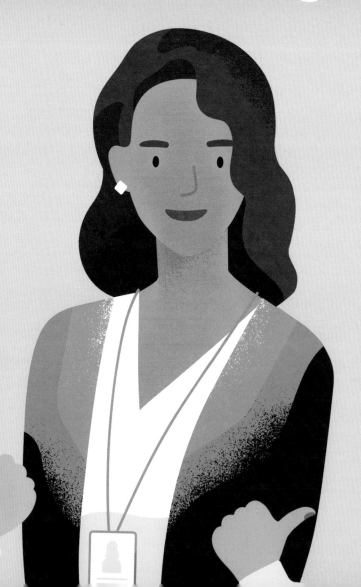

taking
STOCK

What accomplishment are you most proud of?

_____

_____

_____

_____

_____

What makes you proud of it?

_____

_____

_____

_____

What does it say about you?

_____

_____

_____

_____

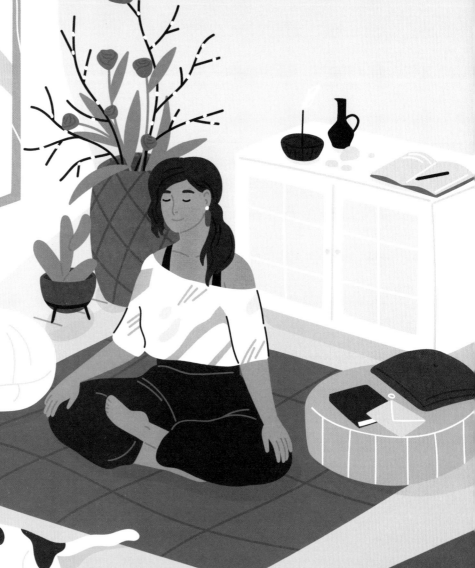

being

PRESENT

What events in your life do you regret not being "present" for (i.e., you were distracted while they were happening)?

_____

_____

_____

_____

_____

_____

_____

_____

_____

What were you doing instead?

_____

_____

_____

What future events will you regret most
if you miss them?

_____

_____

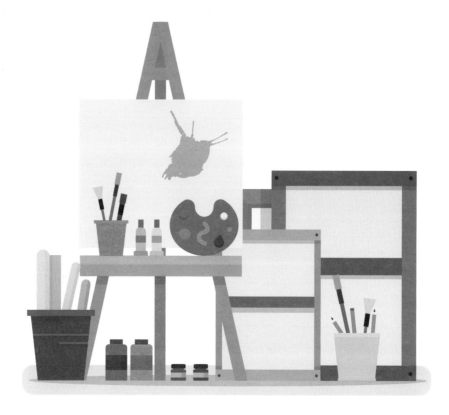

fostering CREATIVITY

What artistic pursuits do you most enjoy?

_____

_____

How do they bring joy to your life?

_____

_____

_____

_____

_____

_____

What are some ways you can nurture your creativity?

_____

_____

_____

_____

_____

_____

_____

_____

time
MANAGEMENT

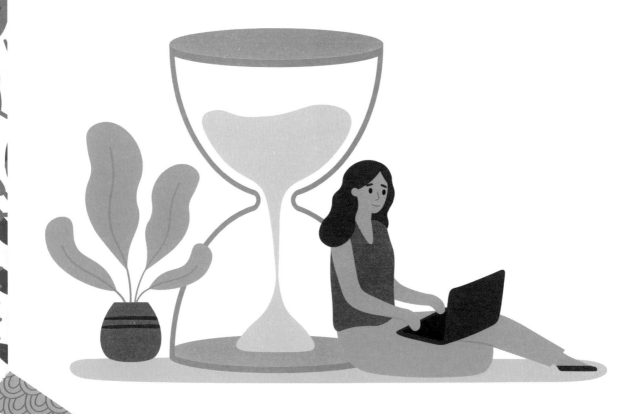

What are the biggest "time bandits" in your life?

_____
_____
_____
_____
_____

What would you rather spend more time on?

_____
_____
_____
_____
_____
_____

What changes could you make to carve out
more time for what's important to you?

_____
_____
_____

your future PERFECT

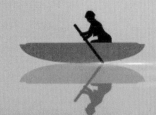

What's your 10-year plan? What do you want
to accomplish? Where will you be living? What will you
be doing? What will be making you happy?

_____

_____

_____

_____

_____

_____

_____

_____

_____

_____

_____

_____

_____

_____

_____

_____

_____

getting it
ALL OUT

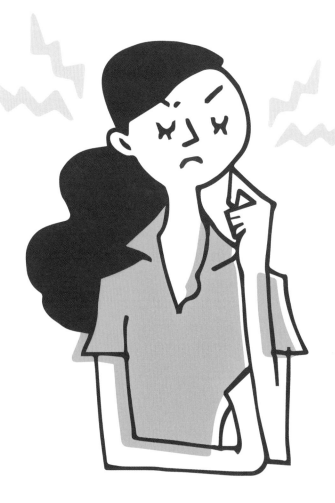

What's your biggest problem right now? Go ahead and vent—what are the circumstances and whose fault is it?

_____

_____

_____

_____

Is there a way to move forward?
What would that look like?

_____

_____

_____

_____

_____

_____

_____

_____

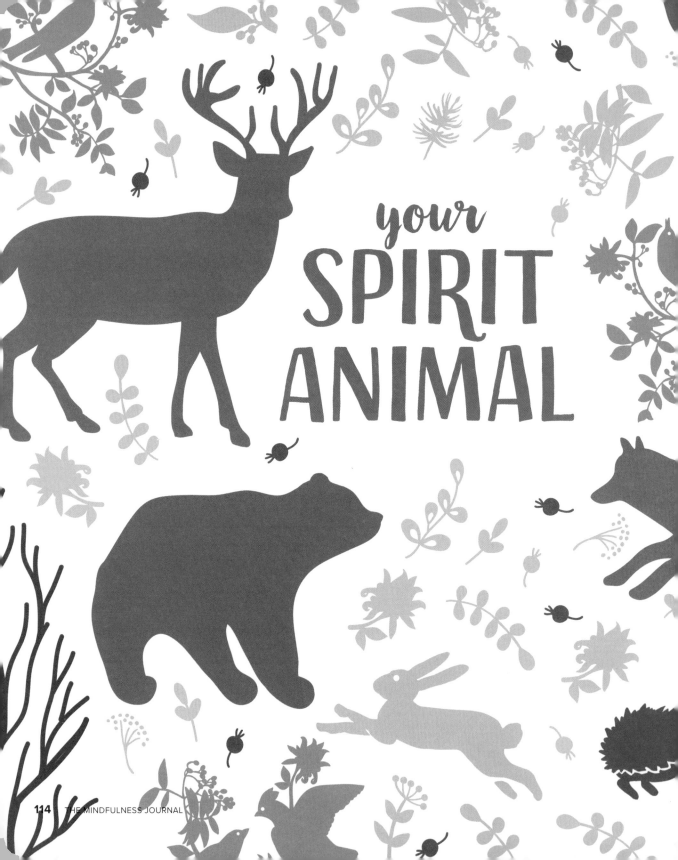

your
SPIRIT
ANIMAL

What is your spirit animal?

_____
_____
_____
_____
_____
_____

What qualities of that animal do you
embody (loyalty, strength, speed, sociability)?

_____
_____
_____

Why do you admire that animal?

_____
_____
_____
_____
_____

your PERSONAL TIME LINE

> "LIFE IS NOT A PROBLEM TO BE SOLVED, BUT A REALITY TO BE EXPERIENCED."
> SØREN KIERKEGAARD

Make a time line of your life—list the 10 most significant events (good and bad) in your life.

1 _____

2 _____

3 _____

4 _____

5 _____

6 _____

7 _____

8 _____

9 _____

10 _____

How did they make you feel?
_____

_____

_____

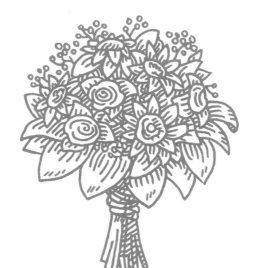

expressing GRATITUDE

"IF YOU CONCENTRATE ON WHAT YOU DON'T HAVE, YOU WILL NEVER, EVER HAVE ENOUGH."

OPRAH WINFREY

What five things are you most grateful for?

_____

_____

_____

_____

_____

_____

_____

How is your life better than it was a year ago?

_____

_____

_____

_____

_____

_____

What personal qualities are you most grateful for?

_____

_____

_____

_____

get
HAPPY

Which five people make you happiest?

1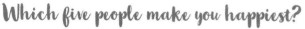

2

3

4

5

What five activities make you happiest?

1 _____

2 _____

3 _____

4 _____

5 _____

What things make you unhappiest?

_____

_____

_____

_____

_____

_____

_____

_____

_____

dear ME

"DESTINY...IS NOT A THING TO BE WAITED FOR, IT IS A THING TO BE ACHIEVED."
WILLIAM JENNINGS BRYAN

Write a letter to your younger self. Pick an age that was especially confusing or upsetting for you. Alleviate the fears you had then, and inspire yourself about what the future holds.

the power of
KINDNESS

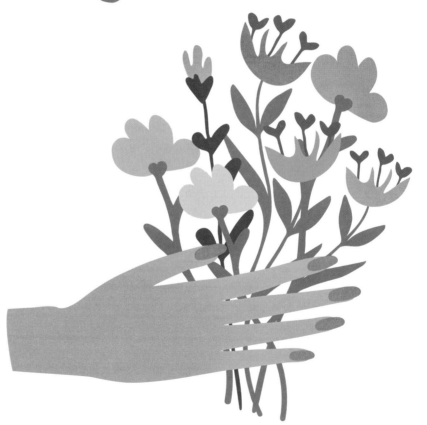

What impact can kindness have on the world?

_____
_____
_____
_____
_____
_____

Make a kindness resolution—how can you be kinder in the future?

_____
_____
_____

How can it change your life?

_____
_____
_____
_____

your
BEST LIFE

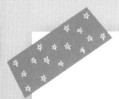

We are often told to live every day as if it's our last day on Earth. If today were the last day of your life, what would you do, from morning to evening?

_____

_____

_____

_____

_____

_____

_____

_____

_____

_____

_____

_____

_____

_____

_____

_____

_____

SELF-PORTRAITS

A SELF-PORTRAIT CAN HELP US SEE OURSELVES MORE CLEARLY.
WHILE YOU CAN DRAW FROM A SELFIE OR WHILE LOOKING IN A
MIRROR, IT'S BEST TO DO IT FREEHAND, FROM MEMORY.

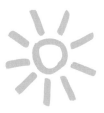

Draw a self-portrait
of yourself as a
CHILD

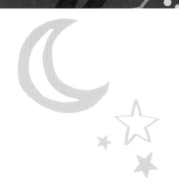

Draw a self-portrait
of yourself as a

TEENAGER

Draw a self-portrait of yourself at this
MOMENT

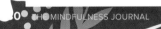

Draw a self-portrait
of yourself in the
FUTURE

COLORING PAGES

ADULTS ARE DISCOVERING WHAT KINDERGARTEN TEACHERS HAVE KNOWN FOR GENERATIONS: COLORING IS A GREAT WAY TO QUIET THE MIND AND CALM THE SPIRIT.

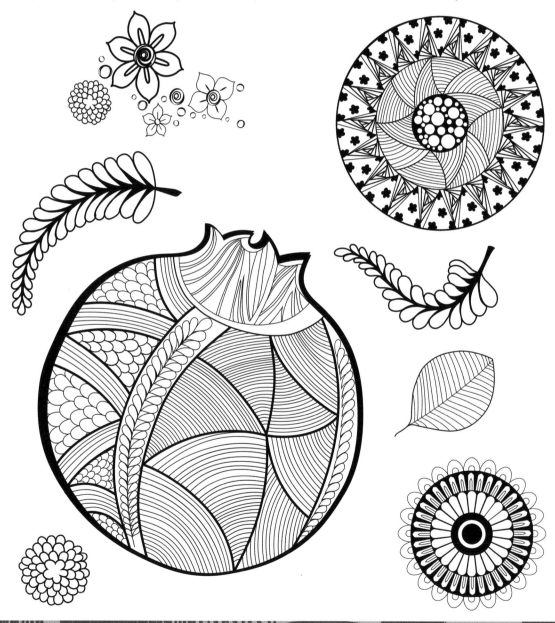

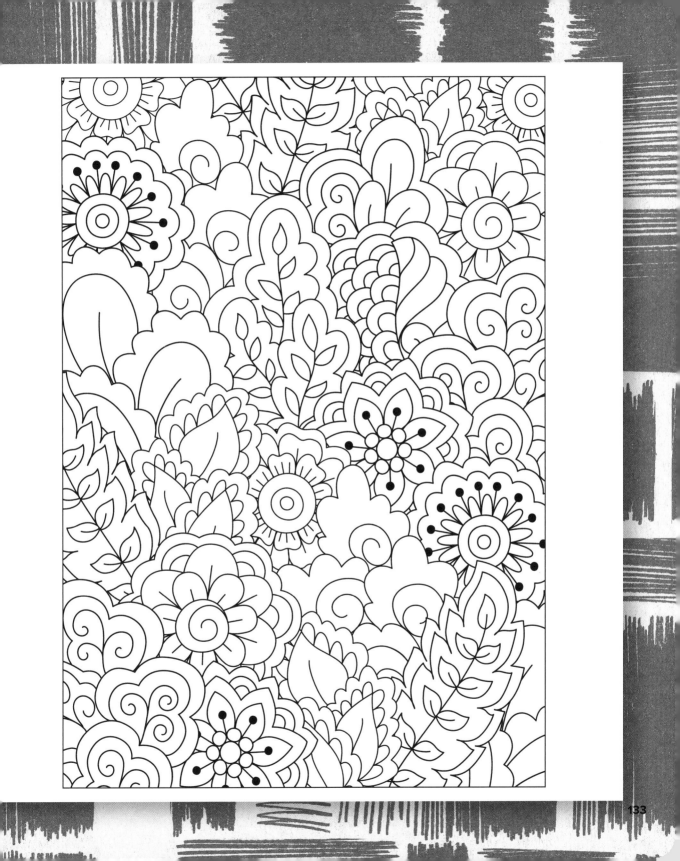

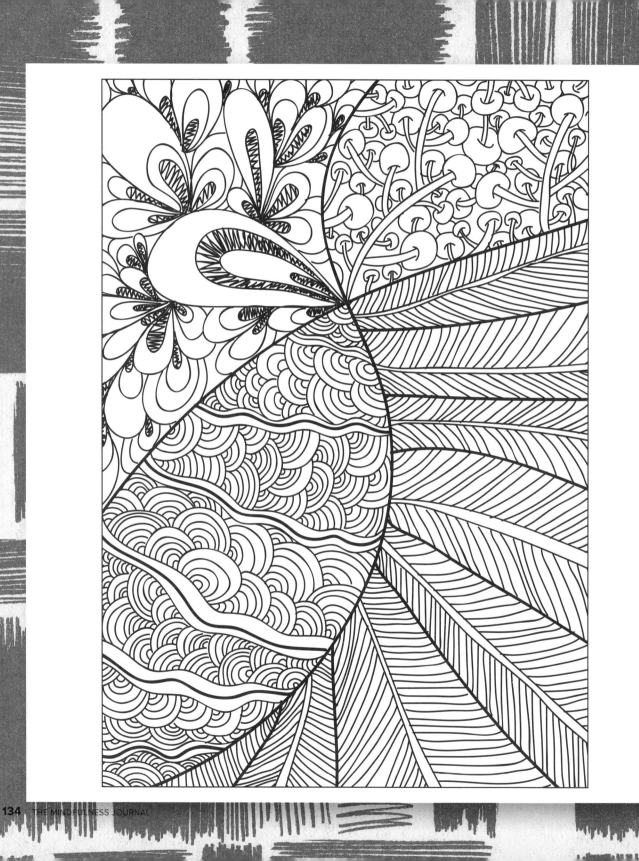

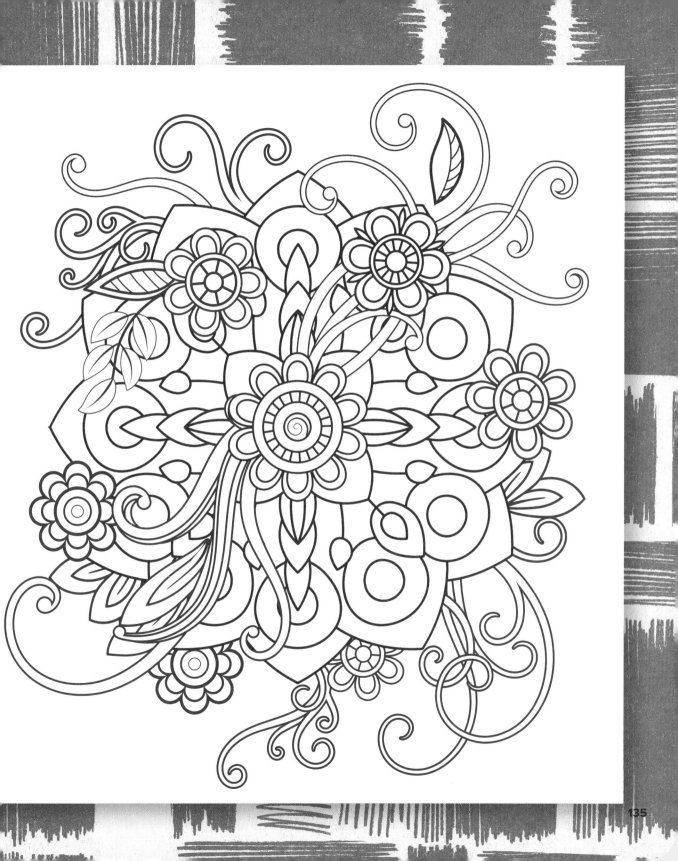

MINDFUL DOODLING

IT MAY SEEM CHILDLIKE, BUT DRAWING SQUIGGLES AND CURLICUES CAN
ACTUALLY BE A FORM OF THERAPY, HELPING YOU RELAX AND DE-STRESS.

doodle a
pattern using
DOTS

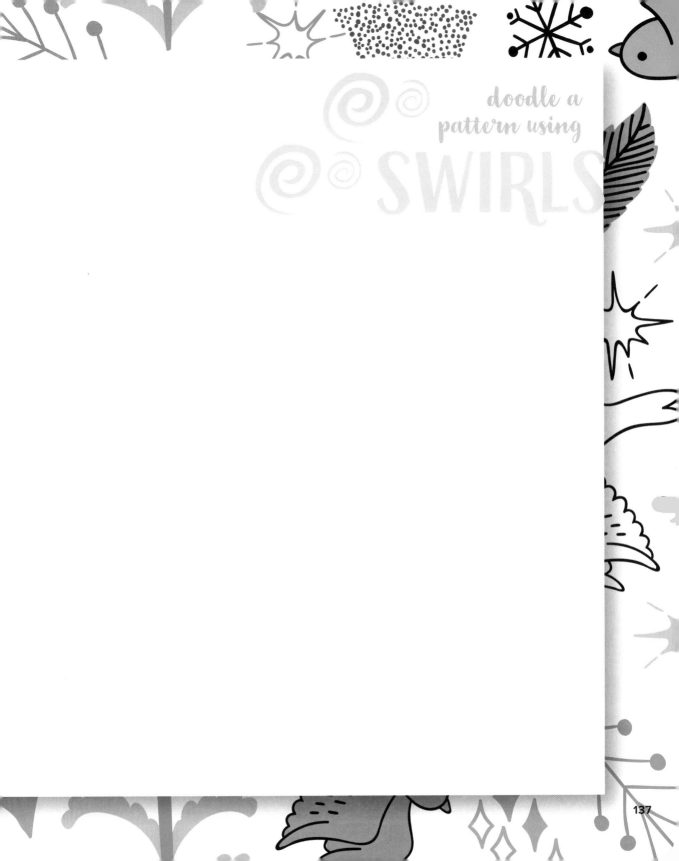

doodle a
pattern using
SWIRLS

doodle a
pattern using
STRAIGHT
LINES

doodle a
pattern using
CIRCLES

INDEX

SPECIAL THANKS TO CONTRIBUTING WRITERS

Amanda Altman, Stacy Baker, Sandra Fernandez, Tess Ghilaga, Beth Johnson, Hallie Levine, Laurie Sprague, Michelle Stacey, Katherine Wessling

Cover Trina Dalziel/Getty Images **2-3** Trina Dalziel/Getty Images **4-5** Clockwise from bottom left: cosmaa/Getty Images; pixelfit/Getty Images; Corey Jenkins/Getty Images; Nata Bene/Shutterstock; Tartila/Shutterstock **6-7** wundervisuals/Getty Images **8-9** pixelfit/Getty Images **11** andresr/Getty Images **12-13** PeopleImages/Getty Images; VeenaMari/Getty Images **14-15** Clockwise from top left: VeenaMari/ Getty Images; PeopleImages/Getty Images; Westend61/Getty Images **16-17** Westend61/Getty Images **19** MmeEmil/Getty Images **20-21** VeenaMari/Getty Images; Max4e Photo/Shutterstock **22-23** Kaspars Grinvalds/Shutterstock **25** Kaspars Grinvalds/Shutterstock **26-27** Clockwise from top left: VeenaMari/ Getty Images; Nongnuch Leelaphasuk/Getty Images; Denys Prykhodov/Shutterstock **29** PeopleImages/ Getty Images **31** VeenaMari/Getty Images **33** kupicoo/Getty Images **34-35** Geber86/Getty Images; VeenaMari/Getty Images **36-37** Sunkids/Shutterstock **39** Corey Jenkins/Getty Images **40-41** Jessica Peterson/Getty Images **43** PeopleImages/Getty Images **44** Africa Studio//Shutterstock **46-47** Teeramet Thanomkiat/Getty Images **48-49** annebaek/Getty Images; VeenaMari/Getty Images **51** PeopleImages/ Getty Images **52-53** Westend61/Getty Images; VeenaMari/Getty Images; Fancy/Getty Images **56-57** Aliyev Alexei Sergeevich/Getty Images; VeenaMari/Getty Images **58-59** Nata Bene/Shutterstock **60** Lumina Images/Getty Images **62-63** VeenaMari/Getty Images; PeopleImages/Getty Images; Hill Street Studios/Getty Images **66-67** SDI Productions/Getty Images; VeenaMari/Getty Images; RossHelen/ Shutterstock **71** istetiana/Getty Images **72, 75** cosmaa/Getty Images **76-77** cosmaa/Getty Images; VeenaMari/Getty Images **78-79** cosmaa/Getty Images; Tom Merton/Getty Images **80-81** Elizaveta Ruzanova/Shutterstock; VeenaMari/Getty Images **82-83** Magnia/Shutterstock; GoodStudio/Shutterstock **84-85** From left: GoodStudio/Shutterstock; sasimoto/Shutterstock; saemilee/Getty Images **86-87** tn-prints/Shutterstock; Marina Malades/Shutterstock; saemilee/Getty Images; sasimoto/Shutterstock **88-89** LuFei/Shutterstock; sasimoto/Shutterstock; Zaie/Shutterstock **90-91** From left: le adhiz/ Shutterstock; cosmaa/Shutterstock; saemilee/Getty Images **92-93** From left: Elena Melnikova/ Shutterstock; sasimoto/Shutterstock; gmark1/Shutterstock; saemilee/Getty Images **94-95** From left: Kaidash_a/Shutterstock; sasimoto/Shutterstock; saemilee/Getty Images **96-97** Maria_Galybina/ Shutterstock; GoodStudio/Shutterstock; sasimoto/Shutterstock; saemilee/Getty Images **98-99** From left: GoodStudio/Shutterstock; sasimoto/Shutterstock; saemilee/Getty Images 100-101 From left: Kaidash_a/ Shutterstock; sasimoto/Shutterstock; Tartila/Shutterstock; saemilee/Getty Images **102-103** From left: GoodStudio/Shutterstock; sasimoto/Shutterstock; saemilee/Getty Images **104-105** From left: GoodStudio/· Shutterstock; sasimoto/Shutterstock **106-107** From left: Irtsya/Shutterstock; sasimoto/Shutterstock; Elvetica/Shutterstock; saemilee/Getty Images **108-109** From left: aria_Galybina/Shutterstock; Tartila/ Shutterstock; saemilee/Getty Images **110-111** From left: krissikunterbunt/Shutterstock; sasimoto/ Shutterstock; saemilee/Getty Images **112-113** From left: Kaidash_a/Shutterstock; hisa_nishiya/ Shutterstock; saemilee/Getty Images **114-115** From left: Yudina Anna/Shutterstock; sasimoto/ Shutterstock; saemilee/Getty Images **116-117** From left: Lera Efremova/Shutterstock; Ladzha/ Shutterstock; sasimoto/Shutterstock; saemilee/Getty Images **118-119** Clockwise from bottom left: Rusanovska/Getty Images; sasimoto/Shutterstock **120-121** From left: Holly Jones/Shutterstock; Jutta Kuss/ Getty Images; sasimoto/Shutterstock; saemilee/Getty Images **122-123** From left: Olian_Rosa/ Shutterstock; sasimoto/Shutterstock **124-125** From left: Alina Sagirova/Shutterstock; sasimoto/ Shutterstock; Nnena Irina/Shutterstock; saemilee/Getty Images **126-127** From left: Shafran/Shutterstock; sasimoto/Shutterstock; saemilee/Getty Images **128-131** unicornbacon/Shutterstock (2) **132-133** CSA Images/Getty Images; Anja Vecta/Shutterstock; Cerama_ama/Shutterstock **134-135** CSA Images/Getty Images; vestenskov/Getty Images; Elinorka/Shutterstock **136-139** Maria_Galybina/Shutterstock (2)

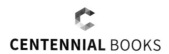

CENTENNIAL BOOKS

An Imprint of
Centennial Media, LLC
40 Worth St., 10th Floor
New York, NY 10013, U.S.A.

ISBN 978-1-951274-19-1
Distributed by
Simon & Schuster, Inc.
1230 Avenue of the Americas
New York, NY 10020, U.S.A.

For information about custom editions, special sales and premium and corporate purchases,
please contact Centennial Media at contact@centennialmedia.com.

Manufactured in China

Publishers & Co-Founders Ben Harris, Sebastian Raatz
Editorial Director Annabel Vered
Creative Director Jessica Power
Executive Editor Janet Giovanelli
Deputy Editors Ron Kelly, Alyssa Shaffer
Design Director Ben Margherita
Art Directors Natali Suasnavas, Joseph Ulatowski
Production Manager Paul Rodina
Production Assistant Alyssa Swiderski
Editorial Assistant Tiana Schippa
Sales & Marketing Jeremy Nurnberg